A Prescription for Psychiatry

*Also by Peter Kinderman*

NEW LAWS OF PSYCHOLOGY: Why Nature and Nurture Alone Cannot Explain Human Behaviour

# A Prescription for Psychiatry

## Why We Need a Whole New Approach to Mental Health and Wellbeing

Peter Kinderman
*University of Liverpool, UK*

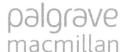

First published 2014 by
PALGRAVE MACMILLAN

Palgrave Macmillan in the UK is an imprint of Macmillan Publishers Limited, registered in England, company number 785998, of Houndmills, Basingstoke, Hampshire RG21 6XS.

Palgrave Macmillan in the US is a division of St Martin's Press LLC, 175 Fifth Avenue, New York, NY 10010.

Palgrave Macmillan is the global academic imprint of the above companies and has companies and representatives throughout the world.

Palgrave® and Macmillan® are registered trademarks in the United States, the United Kingdom, Europe and other countries.

ISBN: 978–1–137–40869–3 Hardback
ISBN: 978–1–137–40870–9 Paperback

This book is printed on paper suitable for recycling and made from fully managed and sustained forest sources. Logging, pulping and manufacturing processes are expected to conform to the environmental regulations of the country of origin.

A catalogue record for this book is available from the British Library.

Library of Congress Cataloging-in-Publication Data

Kinderman, Peter, author.
    A prescription for psychiatry : why we need a whole new approach to mental health and wellbeing / Peter Kinderman.
        p. ; cm.
    Includes bibliographical references.
    ISBN 978–1–137–40869–3 (hardback) – ISBN 978–1–137–40870–9 (paperback)
        I. Title. [DNLM: 1. Health Care Reform. 2. Mental Health Services – organization & administration. 3. Mental Disorders – therapy. 4. Mental Health. 5. Psychiatry – methods. WM 30.1]
RC455
362.2—dc23                                                     2014022080

# Contents

# Acknowledgements

I would like to thank everybody with whom I have shared ideas about this book, and who have helped me by reading and commenting upon earlier drafts. In particular, I would like to thank members of my family, who have been both insightful and patient, and who have helped me enormously in expressing my ideas appropriately. I would also like to thank those colleagues who have helped with more specific advice and help, including Sophie Wilcockson, Joanna Moncrieff and Tim Wilson. I am, of course, enormously grateful to Nicola Jones and all at Palgrave Macmillan who have helped make this book possible. Finally, I would like to express my huge gratitude to Anne Cooke for her enormously helpful contribution to the writing process.

# Introduction: The Disease Model of Mental Health: A System in Crisis

*Traditional thinking about mental health care is profoundly flawed, and radical remedies are required. Our present approach to helping people in acute emotional distress is severely hampered by old-fashioned and incorrect ideas about the nature and origins of mental health problems, and vulnerable people suffer as a result of inappropriate treatment. We must move away from the 'disease model', which assumes that emotional distress is merely a symptom of biological illness, and instead embrace a psychological and social approach to mental health and well-being that recognises our essential and shared humanity.*

Jacqui Dillon is a writer and campaigner on mental health issues. She has both personal and professional experience of working with trauma and abuse, dissociation, 'psychosis', hearing voices, healing and recovery.[1] Jacqui's autobiography – the 'Tale of an Ordinary Little Girl' – tells of how she had '…the misfortune to be born to parents who [were] simply unable to provide the most basic necessities…to be fed and to be kept warm and safe.' She describes a terrible but sadly not uncommon childhood where she '… inhabits a dual world. In one, she is a normal child with normal parents, a gifted child who goes to school, plays with her friends, and likes wearing ribbons in her hair. In the other world, she is a dirty little bitch, evil and unlovable, treated with cruelty and contempt by anyone who can get their filthy hands on her….' Unsurprisingly, Jacqui suffers as a result, and starts hearing voices, '… voices that talk to her, talk about her, who comfort her, protect her and make her feel less alone. In time, they control and terrorise her but help her to stay alive'. When Jacqui herself becomes a mother, she describes how she '…becomes convinced that someone will try and hurt her and her baby because she knows how dangerous the world can be for little

1

children. She becomes intensely fearful; terrified to leave the house in case someone tries to abduct them and take them to the underworld to kill them. She fears that she is going mad like she always knew she would, like they always said she would. She inhabits a dual world....'
In time, understandably, Jacqui turns to the mental health services for help. 'She hopes to find safety and support for her and her precious child and believes that asking for help is a responsible and wise act.' But instead '...to her astonishment, they reiterate the words of the devil.... She is crazy. She is ill. She was born with something wrong with her. She feels as if she has been slapped in the face, kicked while she is down, re-abused. This is insult to injury. She is wild with outrage and has to restrain herself so as not to rip them all to shreds. This reality is enough to drive anyone crazy. The place that is meant to provide her with sanctuary is the place that nearly drives her over the edge once and for all.'
The subject matter of this book – mental health and well-being – is a big topic. We all feel anxious or depressed or confused from time to time, and we certainly all know of people close to us who have had major challenges in their mental health. Throughout history, in literature and politics, we can see the impact of events on the mental health and emotional lives of leaders and citizens alike, and how their decisions, in turn, have been influenced by their psychological well-being. Our mental health and well-being are political and economic issues. The World Health Organization has concluded that mental health problems are the world's leading cause of disability and cost an estimated $2,500 billion worldwide in 2010.[2] Mental health issues have been estimated as costing the UK economy as much as £105 billion each year. In the UK, around 6,000 people take their own lives each year, and (partly as a result of advances in the treatment of infection) the most common cause of death in women in the first year after childbirth is now suicide. This is a large, complex and important issue.

All generalisations are dangerous. Generalisations about mental health care are particularly dangerous, and so are generalisations about any of the professions involved in mental health care, including psychiatry. For every conceivable problem, there are as many different explanations, and possible solutions, as there are individuals on the planet. For every opinion, stance or discipline, there is a diametrically opposed perspective. As we shall see, even within contemporary psychiatry there are opposing traditions and opinions, and there are several different ideas for how best to move forward. For every example, there is a counter-example. But, in my opinion, there are still old-fashioned and unscientific ideas about the nature and origins of mental health problems, meaning that much of mental health care remains dominated (albeit subtly) by a psychiatric 'disease-model' approach. Taking its lead from physical health care, our mental health care system applies 'diagnoses' to emotional, behavioural and psychological issues – most psychiatrists diagnose 'mental illnesses'. Once illnesses are diagnosed, people's life experiences and their views on the origin of their problems are often unfortunately seen as effectively irrelevant. Adopting the medical perspective, the 'aetiologies' (causes) of those supposed 'illnesses' are investigated – with the assumption, of course, that this way of thinking is appropriate. And then, 'treatments' are prescribed. If, on the other hand, an illness isn't diagnosed, it is difficult – perhaps impossible – to receive help. The assumption is that, if there's no illness, there is no problem. All this means that vulnerable people, people in acute emotional distress, frequently suffer.

Various pressures conspire to maintain this system. For many professionals – clinical psychologists as well as psychiatrists – there is little mileage in changing a system that gives them employment, status and power (in some cases a very great deal of status and power). For professionals who lead or manage services, traditional approaches to mental health care maintain the status quo. This is, of course, particularly true for those who are in positions of the greatest power, status, and salary and would therefore apply most to psychiatrists. But the traditional 'disease model' benefits other people too. When a person's problems are described as symptoms of 'an illness', it changes the way we think about personal responsibility. This is why many campaigns aimed at reducing stigma and discrimination against people with mental health problems tend to stress the medical model (using slogans such as 'mental illness is as real as a broken arm'). If – it is argued – we stop seeing a person as feckless, inadequate, evil, possessed by demons, criminally recidivist or wilfully difficult, then we might have a little more sympathy. And – this argument goes – it is therefore helpful to see a person as 'ill'. The problems with this point of view are numerous. Unfortunately, people are often sufficiently illogical as to see people as *both* ill and feckless, which actually increases stigma. And unfortunately for this argument, people are frequently very stigmatising and discriminatory against people identified as having illnesses (think of AIDS, cancer, learning difficulties, sexually-transmitted infections or leprosy). Identifying the various expressions of personal distress as 'symptoms of mental illness' change the way we think about personal responsibility, and that makes the 'disease model' attractive. It means we can argue for sympathy, and at the same time it locates the problems within the individual. And *that* means that we don't have to harbour uncomfortable thoughts about the human cost of war, domestic abuse, rape, the sexual abuse of children, unemployment, poverty, loneliness and failure. All these troubling issues – the factors that can lead us all to become distressed – can be kept comfortably at arm's length.

Most importantly, the 'disease-model' approach to mental health is attractive to pharmaceutical companies. There is a very healthy market for psychiatric drugs. In the UK, each year, we spend £800m on psychoactive drugs. So we can see a rather complex, cynical system conspiring to support the 'disease model'. Social problems with very understandably distressing consequences are sidelined, and indeed the individual problems themselves are glossed over. Instead, the focus of attention moves to so-called 'mental illnesses'. Conveniently for those with vested interests in the current system, the 'illness' idea shifts attention away from the social causes. With the problems labelled as 'illnesses', we now focus on looking for pathologies within the individual – whether genetic or biological abnormalities, or 'thinking errors'. An expensive system develops to 'treat' these 'illnesses', with all the professional consequences. And the multinational pharmaceutical companies step in to offer drugs – at a profit.

This 'disease model' underpins too much of modern mental health care. In my experience, it often strips professionals of their ability to empathise. Because the patient's behaviour is seen as irrational, the product of an 'illness', even a disease, we stop trying to understand the human reasons why they might be feeling or acting the way they are. This is horrible. When people are experiencing huge distress and feel that their sanity, even their life, is threatened, they need empathy and compassion more than ever. That requires understanding human behaviour and distress in a whole new way. It also means we need to plan the delivery of mental health services in completely different ways.

This is a book about mental health care and about social support for mental well-being. It proposes a radical, social and psychological model of care. And yet its title refers to 'a prescription for psychiatry'. The implications of the message in this book extend beyond one profession, and yet I think it is reasonable to highlight one profession in the title. While this is a manifesto for a 'psychobiosocial model', the dominance of medical thinking in this area is such that the word 'psychiatry' is used interchangeably with the term 'mental healthcare' – much to the annoyance of people like myself in non-medical professions. And perhaps there is more to be changed in respect to this medical perspective. My intention, however, in choosing a title was not to target psychiatry and to label that one profession as the root of all evil. It was chosen because of the current dominance of that profession in the field, and because it's the term most people use. Now is a good time for us to rethink the basic principles both of how we understand problems and how we provide services. In response to the American Psychiatric Association's latest version of its diagnostic manual – DSM-5 – in 2013, which I will discuss in more detail in Chapter 2, the British Psychological Society called for a 'paradigm change' in our thinking.[3] I have a few personal credentials for this task. I'm a practising clinical psychologist, and have seen these issues in my day-to-day work. I've twice been Chair of my professional body (the British Psychological Society's Division of Clinical Psychology) and have been involved as a policy-maker in many of these debates. I'm currently a line-manager of psychiatrists, psychologists, nurses, public health doctors and GPs. I am the sibling of someone with serious mental health problems and I've seen how help from mental health professionals can be life-saving but also how the mental health system can cause untold misery to someone who is already suffering. And I've been a personal user of mental health services: I received NHS psychotherapy from a medical (psychiatric) psychotherapist for two years.

## '... you'll need some running shoes...'

We all have nightmares from time to time. The dark, early, hours of the morning are full of various terrors. Mine have always included the idea that I might be detained on a secure psychiatric ward. I know I could rage and fulminate or even attempt to escape, but I'd be overpowered, sedated and restrained. I could argue with the nurses and try to persuade them that I'm fine to go home, but from personal experience I'm pretty sure they'd simply ignore me. Rather depressingly, I'm forced to conclude that the best way to get out of my nightmare would be to go along with the system. This exact scenario, in fact, was the topic of a recent blog[4] which outlined three options for escape: 'the runner' ('you'll need some running shoes, a good hiding place'), 'play the game' ('you'll need good acting skills, some knowledge of psychiatry') and 'the Tribunal' ('you'll need a solicitor').

Back in 1973, David Rosenhan conducted a now-celebrated study into the invalidity of psychiatric diagnosis.[5] He arranged for eight ordinary people from conventional backgrounds to present themselves to a number of psychiatrists at hospitals in the USA. In each case the individuals complained of hearing disembodied voices saying 'empty', 'hollow' or 'thud'. Apart from complaining of this distressing 'symptom' (which, of course, was intended to resemble what conventional wisdom regards as 'hallucinations') the eight undercover researchers were told to answer all questions honestly. Published with the title 'on being sane in insane places', the research reported how all eight individuals were admitted to psychiatric hospitals, in most cases with a diagnosis of schizophrenia. Despite behaving entirely normally after admission, the researchers remained in hospital for an average of 19 days (with a range of seven to 52), during which time they were prescribed a total of 2,100 pills (that's 260 pills each, or 14 per day). The undercover reporters took careful notes of their experiences – and it is interesting that this behaviour was also interpreted as obsessional and pathological. Rosenhan's research has been criticised. It is perhaps fair to point out that it is reasonable to offer help – even medical help – to someone who reports that they are hearing auditory hallucinations and are becoming distressed. One criticism of this research is that it's hard to come to valid and reliable diagnoses if the 'pseudo-patient' in front of you is lying (the researchers were, of course, guilty of faking their experiences). But it is nevertheless shocking that, once admitted, nothing resembling real care was offered. It is important and interesting, for example, that staff members only spent 11% of their time interacting with patients, and that comments like 'Come on, you mother f – – -s, get out of bed' were reported as common. Despite the prescription of 2,100 pills, daily contacts with psychiatrists, psychologists and nurses totalled only seven minutes.

It could be argued that this is a historical account; that things are better now than in 1973. Which is probably true. But not much better. The client of a colleague of mine had been admitted to an in-patient psychiatric ward under a section of the Mental Health Act in response to her quite distressing self-harm. Because she would take pretty much every opportunity to harm herself, she was under constant observation by nurses. This observation extended to accompanying her to a physical care ward to have her wounds attended to (where, incidentally, the nurse told her that she was 'just there to observe, not to talk to you') and to her mother's funeral. On returning from the funeral, a vase of flowers from her mother's memorial service was removed from her room. The rationale given to her was that her 'bad behaviour' would be punished by their removal and her 'good behaviour' rewarded with their return. This is as crazy as it is callous; if the woman was considered to be able to control her behaviour by sheer force of will, surely she shouldn't be detained and observed on a secure psychiatric ward. And if she were ill, insane, and unable to control her behaviour, why would the contingencies of reward and punishment make any difference? It seems as if the presumption is that the pain of the punitive treatment needs to be severe enough to penetrate to the mind of the insane patient. We can see some of the ways in which the 'disease-model' ways of thinking can lead to quite callous approaches when we see 'observation' in mental health care settings. It's not uncommon for people who report hearing voices, or that they have had thoughts of harming and even killing themselves to be placed under 'observation'. Not very much therapeutically is actually done, but the person is 'observed', and prevented from harming themselves. The underlying assumption seems to be that the voices or the suicidal thoughts are the result of an illness, and the client needs to be kept under observation while that illness is being treated. Perhaps the most striking example of this that I came across was when I was asked to write a commentary for a book chapter describing clinical dilemmas on an in-patient psychiatric ward. In brief, the case involved a woman who was very distressed and agitated. She was described as experiencing a 'manic episode'. As I read the description, the story became both very clear and rather disturbing. The clinical dilemma was written from the perspective of persuading her to take medication. While nursing or medical staff were sitting with her and talking with her about her various (admittedly rather incoherent) concerns, she was described as being relatively calm. Whenever the subject of medication was raised, or if the nurses suggested that they might have to leave, she would become very distressed. The account ended with a rather heartfelt description of how the staff felt that they had no option but to force medication on her; a very distressing experience. I remember being struck by the contrast between the medical approach – the principled feeling that the client needed to receive the medicine that would help her – and my own feeling that, since she seemed to be comforted by having a professional sitting with her and listening, then that should continue, for hours if necessary, until sleep offered respite. The contrast in assumptions seemed striking to me.

More personally, I remember vising a psychiatric hospital to see a relative a few years ago (at that point receiving in-patient care). We were sitting on or near his bed, and a fellow patient shuffled past. My relative gave him a friendly greeting, but the other patient offered little more than a grunt in reply. I asked if he was OK, and my relative replied that his friend had received ECT earlier that day, and was still a little groggy. I then made a rather foolish mistake; I asked if it was 'working'. My relative looked at me, wrinkled his nose, smiled in a sardonic kind of way, stroked his beard and said: 'Well... He came in here a few days ago and told them he was depressed. They electrocuted his head; what do you think he'll tell them now?' My point isn't really to discuss the effectiveness and ethics of ECT, although I fear the side effects outweigh any benefits, the benefits may in fact be close to non-existent, and I would not include ECT in my prescription for an ethical service. My point is that many people, including my relative, experience the mental health care system – dominated by a 'disease-model' ideology – as punitive, oppressive and punishing.

It might be hard for those charged with responsibility to hear this, but standards of care in many mental healthcare clinics are disgraceful. I receive a fair number of unsolicited letters. One summed up the situation nicely: ' ... *Rather than engaging with the patients on the ward, the staff instead shepherded them around like sheep with bullying commands, threats of 'jabs' (injections), and removal to an acute ward elsewhere in the hospital, if they did not co-operate. The staff also stressed medication rather than engagement as a way of controlling the patients. And the staff closeted themselves in the ward office, instead of being out and about on the corridors and in the vestibule where they should have been. The staff wrote daily reports on each patient on the hospital's Intranet system; these reports were depended upon by the consultant psychiatrists for their diagnoses and medication prescriptions, but were patently fabricated and false, because the staff had never engaged or observed properly the patient they were writing about in their reports. The psychiatrists themselves were rarely seen on the ward, and only consulted with their patients once a week.'*

I believe that the care offered to people with mental health problems in the UK is amongst the best in the world. But rather sadly that merely points out how bad it must be elsewhere. Caring people would, I think, agree that we should encourage all nations to invest appropriately in mental health care. Until recently, Britain had a good record here. We spend around 10% of our (substantial) GDP on healthcare; a figure which has risen steadily (although that's recently reported to have dropped very slightly).[6] In general we spend that investment efficiently (because we have the NHS). And we spend a relatively high proportion (around 12%) of that healthcare budget on mental health (5.5% is the European average). That's all good, but it doesn't look as if the investment is paying dividends in terms of high quality care and greater well-being. Although my hard-working colleagues will regard my words as undermining their efforts, I believe that the care that people receive in both community and residential care settings (I shall try to avoid the terms 'in-patient' and 'out-patient', because I don't think the word 'patient' is appropriate when discussing emotional well-being) falls short of what's expected. In 2011, the independent *Schizophrenia Commission* was established by the charity and pressure-group *Rethink*

*Mental Illness*, and in 2012 published the report 'Schizophrenia – The Abandoned Illness'.[7] Among other recommendations (which echo many of the calls I'll be making later in this book, for example, calling for greater access to psychological therapies, a right to a second opinion on medication, greater reliance on the skills of pharmacists and general practitioners, etc.) the Commission called for 'a radical overhaul of poor acute care units'.

The Schizophrenia Commission, helpfully reviewing decades of research, suggested that acute residential mental health care (in-patient psychiatric wards) is likely always to be part of the services we provide. The problems faced by people in acute distress mean that community services are unlikely ever to completely replace residential, in-patient, care. But the Commission did not find a happy picture. There has been a plethora of recent guidelines and initiatives in an attempt to refocus and improve the quality of residential care, most notably and recently by the influential NICE, the National Institute of Health and Care Excellence.[8] But residential care remains highly unpopular with service users and carers. There is also a 'shortage of beds'. In the medical language of healthcare, planners like to talk about 'beds' – the resources available are calculated on the basis of how many beds the medical wards have available for patients. I personally fear that even this jargon dehumanises and reminds us that this is a highly medical approach to care. There is a shortage of alternatives, and the services that we do deign to provide are often very stretched. That often has a complex impact, as it means that people are reluctant to enter residential units because of the pressurised and stressful atmosphere. Pressure for 'beds' also means that people are often discharged before their problems are resolved or without proper care having been planned for after their discharge. At the same time, people who could leave hospital if there were appropriate alternative specialist services are often detained for far too long; longer than would be the case if appropriate services were available in the community. On these residential units, there are worrying levels of violence against both staff and service users, sexual harassment, and theft, with drug and alcohol problems common. This is wholly unacceptable. When people are distressed, we need an 'asylum', a place of safety and calm, where we can resolve tension and stress and overcome trauma … not be exposed to abuse and assault. And finally, in this maelstrom of stress, residential units are also plagued by boredom, a lack of purposeful activity, a lack of staff–patient interaction, and inadequate physical environments. Indeed, the Commission Chair, Professor Sir Robin Murray, stated that; 'the message that comes through loud and clear is that people are being badly let down by the system in every area of their lives.'

It's perhaps not too surprising, therefore, that in the UK, our official surveys of the quality of care of in-patient wards explicitly exclude mental health care.[9] Unsurprising, perhaps, because politicians are generally unwilling to encourage publicity of failings in the care systems for which they are responsible, and because traditionally the voices of those seen as 'mentally ill' have been silenced. As I suggested earlier, respectable commentators have suggested that the UK has one of the best mental healthcare systems in the world (at least in 2006)[10] and so we should, we're wealthy enough to afford it. Rather unfortunately, that suggests that people in other countries have much worse provision still.

In the USA, for example, it's widely estimated that until very recently – with the very welcome development of 'Obamacare', which made healthcare insurance mandatory, universal and automatic – some 40% of citizens had no healthcare insurance. Despite 'Obamacare', we're still living with that legacy, meaning that only about half of all people with mental health problems receive any form of planned care. For the rest, there's a mixed picture; from various forms of charitable services through to state mental institutions with poor reputations. America, as is often the case, presents a mixed picture, with very high levels of investment in all forms of mental health care for the wealthy, but also neglect for poor and socially disadvantaged people. There is also an extraordinary range of approaches. It is striking that it was some American techniques for people who have been given a diagnosis of autism that were described by a recent UN report as being 'akin to torture'.[11] The particular techniques that gave such cause for concern involved children wearing special devices that administered electric shocks to modify their behaviour.[12] In the developing world, the picture is again complex. It seems likely that for people who avoid formal psychiatric care, the prognosis is if anything at least as good as in the industrialised world.[13] Formal, institutional, care in much of the developing world is concerning, with disturbing stories of physical restraint, chemical sedation and very poor standards of care.

We need to invest appropriately in mental health care. We need to maintain Britain's enviable record in this respect.[14] But we also need to ensure that our investment is in fact leading to high quality care and ensuring greater well-being.

## A flawed ethos

The work of medically trained psychiatrists is a vital contribution to mental health care. But this doesn't necessarily mean we should assume that people are ill. Pregnancy is a good analogy. Doctors in a variety of specialisms (general practitioners, obstetricians, paediatricians) all offer valuable care for pregnant women. Pregnancy can sometimes have potentially serious medical complications. But pregnancy, itself, is not an illness. Similarly, when a multidisciplinary team offers care to a person in distress, I believe medical colleagues have much to offer. But many aspects of the ethos of 'care' in current, traditional, mental health care are actively harmful – people are effectively told that they are 'ill', and have an underlying biological abnormality. In my opinion, this 'disease model' is scientifically incorrect, inherently illogical and has serious harmful consequences. I believe that this 'disease model' contributes to the negative, punitive, controlling ethos that often prevails in services. It undermines genuine empathy and compassion; instead of seeing people's difficulties as understandable and natural responses to the terrible things that have happened to them, the person is seen as having something wrong with them – an 'illness'.

The 'medical model' of mental health care – the belief that psychological distress has a biological cause, and that mental health problems are essentially medical diseases – is controversial even within psychiatry. 'Social psychiatry' takes a different view to 'biological psychiatry' and has a different view about the future of psychiatry as a discipline. Many psychiatrists (and, indeed, psychologists) feel these terms are misleading or meaningless. Nevertheless, a 'disease model' is ubiquitous. Naturally, the pharmaceutical industry promotes this approach heavily. It makes sense to take a medical drug to 'cure' a medical 'illness'.[15] Some people also find this approach helpful in certain ways – for example it is one way of explaining problems without blaming the person. The problem is that it is misleading.

Firstly, there is only very weak evidence for genetic causes of mental health problems. On a very technical level, much of the evidence used to support a biological model is dubious. The fact that many problems appear to have high 'heritability' – that they tend to 'run in families – does not necessarily imply that there are biological, genetically inherited characteristics at work. I'll illustrate this with two slightly odd – but entirely factual – examples. Because rich people tend to have children who turn out themselves to be rich, and people living in developed countries tend to have children who also live in those countries, car ownership is highly 'heritable'; car ownership runs in families. On the other hand (sorry about the pun), the likelihood of having five fingers (or, to be exact, four fingers and a thumb) on each hand has a statistical 'heritability' close to zero.[16] Despite the spurious correlation that you may find if you search for 'heritability' and 'IQ' or 'mental illness' on the internet, simple biological determinism is difficult to sustain on close examination. It's also almost certainly the case that a very large number of genetic variants all conspire to offer generally increased or decreased risks of a wide variety of problems (rather than 'a gene for X'). At the same time, a very wide variety of injuries and insults to the body and brain (influenza in pregnancy, birth difficulties, injury, drug use etc.) again all conspire in very general ways to increase our risk of developing problems.

Researchers have used a number of techniques to explore genetic influences on mental health and well-being. We have compared identical and non-identical twins, and we have studied the biological and adoptive relatives of people who were subsequently given a diagnosis of a mental health problem. More recently, scientists have begun to use a technique called 'genome-wide association study' or 'GWAS', which is used to look very precisely at genetic differences between people with or without a particular disease.

It is clear that the tendency to experience mental health problems can run in families. But this is not necessarily a result of genetics. It is very difficult to disentangle genetic inheritance from environmental factors such as upbringing and social circumstances. The methodology and results of studies relating to genetic factors in 'schizophrenia', for example, are hotly debated in professional journals. In the early days of genetic research, it was common to discuss the idea of a 'gene for schizophrenia'. Now, it is much more common to discuss more general genetic 'risk'. This means that there may be many heritable characteristics which each increase the likelihood of someone experiencing mental health problems if they are exposed to particular life events.

Modern biological science has given us remarkable insights into the genetics of these phenomena. The findings are both striking and thought-provoking. But it is clear that the picture is much more complex than: '...schizophrenia is a genetic disease...'. Genetic factors play a role in all human phenomena, from voting for political parties to falling in love and aggression, as well as mental health and well-being. The genetic parts of this jigsaw are both common to many different experiences, and also interact with environmental factors, so it is difficult to suggest any one element is more important than any other. Perhaps it's a little like asking: what's more important in a water molecule, hydrogen or oxygen?

It does seem clear that there are (a very large number of) genetic factors that increase the (general) vulnerability or likelihood of people to experience mental health problems. But there is no inevitability, and the genetic factors interact with environmental factors. These genetic factors apply to a wide range of mental health problems – psychosis (hearing voices or experiencing paranoia), mood swings, social communication and difficulties in concentration. Modern approaches to genetics have also highlighted the role of 'epigenetics': the phenomenon whereby important parts of our genetic mechanisms are 'switched on' or moderated by external or environmental factors. So, for instance, a gene that is responsible for the production of a specific protein may be more or less active, and may produce more or less of that protein, in different environmental conditions.

It is fundamentally important to remember this interaction between genes and environment. Imagine a world in which everybody – every single human being without exception – smoked 40 cigarettes a day. The prevalence of lung cancer would, of course, be enormously high. But not everybody would develop lung cancer. Some people would be genetically more vulnerable than others. And – since everybody smokes – these genetic differences would be the only real source of differential risks. The same, incidentally, is true if nobody smoked – again, genetic differences would be important. In the real world today, about 20% of people in the UK smoke cigarettes. And it is whether or not you expose yourself to this massive risk factor that is more important than the degree of your genetic vulnerability. The same seems to be true of mental health. Of course genetic factors are important, but we often ignore the 'elephant in the room' – the environmental causes of distress.

More to the point, there is no reason to assume that any biological 'abnormalities' are necessarily biological causes. We know, as an illustration, that the hippocampus is a physical area of the brain involved in memory. It's fascinating that taxi-drivers' hippocampi physically change as they develop their 'mental maps' of London. That's a physical change in the brain as a result of environmental factors – in that case, learning. It would be ludicrous to suggest that the changes in the brain, in the hippocampus, are unrelated to the taxi-driver learning more about the physical geography of London, but it's equally ludicrous to suggest that the changes in the hippocampus have 'caused' changes in the taxi-driver's behaviour. So brain studies in mental health are vitally important as we struggle to understand ourselves better. But we have to be careful how we interpret them, and in particular not to use biologically reductionist arguments. For instance, there is widespread acceptance that a particular brain chemical called dopamine plays a role in psychosis; but the details are far from clear-cut. Some of the psychological processes involved in psychosis (for example making creative links between apparently unrelated things) appear to use dopamine as a principal neurotrans-mitter. Biological differences between, for example, people who are or are not experiencing psychosis are also small and inconsistent. It is not the case, for instance, that everybody with a diagnosis of schizophrenia shows any particular biological abnormality, most people who receive a diagnosis of 'schizophrenia' report no family history of similar problems, and everybody responds to medication differently. And, in any event, as with taxi-drivers' brains, we know that dopaminergic pathways are influenced by, among other things, abuse and chronic victimisation.[17] Life events and experiences can alter our brain biology.

This is important, because there is evidence that the 'disease model' leads to stigma and discrimination. Many people assume that promoting a biological understanding of mental health problems will reduce stigma. But there is quite strong evidence that the opposite is the case; biological models actually promote stigma. We know that people in receipt of mental health care experience high levels of stigma and discrimination.[18] Traditional attempts to reduce this stigma have – of course – stemmed from the 'disease model', biomedical approach, and have tried to make the case that 'mental illness is an illness like any other'.[19] On the whole, these have had only limited success; negative attitudes towards people with mental health problems seem to have either remained stable over time or even got worse. That's actually hardly surprising. People experience stigma with many physical illnesses such as cancer, AIDS and leprosy. It simply does not follow that to be seen as ill protects a person from stigma… although it seems superficially attractive. In fact, in my opinion the most biological of biological explanations – genetic abnormality – is quintessentially stigmatising. Genetic explanations suggest that people experience difficulties because their genetic blueprint, their DNA, is faulty. If we say that a particular trait is: a) undesirable, and b) part of the most fundamental, heritable (that is, transmissible to the next generation) and immutable genome of the individual, we are clearly associating that person fundamentally with the undesirability. We may well feel some sympathy with someone who is 'ill', but locating an undesirable social phenomenon within the essential nature of a person is also very stigmatising. Although it is entirely possible for psychological models themselves to be stigmatising (they still focus attention on what goes on inside people's heads, rather than on what has happened to them), there is evidence that explaining things in terms of biology tends to lead to greater discrimination.[20] A non-medical approach to understanding and helping is likely to be the most effective in reducing stigma and discrimination.

This all means that, despite enormous volumes of scientific evidence that social factors lead to mental health problems and, consequently, widespread acceptance of the social basis of much of the distress, routine mental health care in practice relies on the attempted treatment of illnesses assumed to reside, physically, in the body (more specifically the brain), as opposed to helping people to address these social challenges. In fact, the dominance of this disease model is so pervasive that sometimes we have to step back before we realise how powerfully it's affecting our thinking. In Liverpool recently, colleagues of mine conducted an elegant analysis of the impact of the economic recession on suicide rates. They concluded that around a thousand people had taken their own lives as a result of the recent financial crisis and recessions – the economic mismanagement of our bankers really is a matter of life and death. My colleagues John Read and Richard Bentall and others[21] have conducted an extensive review of the effects of childhood trauma (abuse) on our mental health. It's kind of obvious... abuse has consequences; trauma is traumatic. There is overwhelming evidence that poor housing, unemployment and social disadvantage of all kinds contribute to mental ill-health.

Interestingly, there's also plenty of evidence that inequalities, both economic and social, are particularly important. In their book 'The Spirit Level', Richard Wilkinson and Kate Pickett argued that, once a nation has achieved a certain basic level of economic performance, the well-being of its citizens is much more closely linked to economic equality than to average economic performance.[22] Wilkinson and Pickett compared a range of successful, industrialised nations (the 'G20' nations) and found that, on a series of measures such as physical health, obesity, substance misuse, education, crime and violence, and (of course) mental health, the greater the difference between the rich and poor, the worse a nation performed.

It's easy to see why this could be the case. Human beings have an innate tendency to compare (it's actually part of the way our neurones work) and comparison between people in terms of material success and all its implications can be invidious for our sense of self-worth. The point is that social and economic factors are – quite understandably – strong predictors of mental health problems. But these social factors are simply squeezed out – the very real, very important, very pressing, social factors that lead to mental health problems are minimised and ignored.

We know that issues such as poverty, deprivation, social isolation, childhood abuse (of various forms) all lead to distress or what are (mis) diagnosed as mental disorders. Systematic research into both social and biological causes of mental health problems has revealed, for example, that the more abuse and deprivation suffered by individuals, the more likely they are to experience psychological or mental health problems. This 'dose–response' effect is hardly surprising... what is surprising is the way that mental health professionals sometimes respond. It is not uncommon, for instance, for quite senior scientists simply to deny that social factors play any role in the origin of, for example, 'schizophrenia'. Then, when the evidence starts to emerge, its impact is minimised or sidelined. Social causes of mental health problems can be turned into consequences – for example unemployment described as a consequence of depression rather than the other way around. And people sometimes seem to go to extreme lengths to fit emerging facts into their existing world-view. For example, one commentator on a recent paper discussing the emotional impact of childhood abuse suggested that: '*the possibility cannot be ruled out that a child destined to develop schizophrenia may show characteristics in childhood that increase the risk of abuse*'.[23] In other words, even if we find that mental health problems are the consequence of abuse... maybe there we can still find genetic abnormalities that ulti- mately put you at risk of abuse! This begins to look slightly self-serving logic, ironically even perhaps delusional.

An alternative take on this theme was reflected in a recent discus- sion about the genetics of 'attention deficit hyperactivity disorder' or 'ADHD'. I recently attended a meeting of (mainly biological) psychia- trists which generated a great deal of heated discussion over the treat- ment of a colleague in the media. It was generally felt that she had been subjected to unwarranted criticism. She had presented what was described as excellent research into the genetics of ADHD – reporting on a statistically significantly greater prevalence of a particular genetic abnormality in children who had received a diagnosis of ADHD. The research had revealed that 16% of children who had been given a diag- nosis of ADHD had a particular genetic variant, in comparison with only 8% of children without the diagnosis.[24] This research had been subjected to considerable criticism (unfairly, in the opinion of those attending my meeting) by opponents of biological psychiatry. I pointed out that Ben Goldacre had explicitly drawn attention to this work in his column 'bad science', because, although the researcher had discovered a statistically significant association, 84% of children with a diagnosis of ADHD did not possess the particular genetic variant at the heart of the research.[25] I suggested that this hardly justified the comment that 'now we can say with confidence that ADHD is a genetic disease', and that the statement was potentially misleading. The response (by colleagues nonplussed by my outburst) was to suggest that she (the quoted researcher) really meant nothing more than that there was a genetic element to ADHD, it didn't mean environmental factors were unimportant. My view is... when a doctor states 'with confidence' that a particular problem is 'a genetic disease', then that's exactly how this kind of statement will be interpreted. And, I have to say, I strongly suspect that this is what some people believe.

This is not just an academic issue. In my view, a strong belief in the 'disease model' of mental health and in the genetic origins of mental health problems, despite lack of evidence, is at least partly responsible for the relentless assault that the system itself seems to inflict on vulnerable people. The enormous weight of evidence showing that people are distressed as a result of the sometimes terrible and sometimes just miserable things that happen to them appears not to permeate into care. A profound change is needed both in the way we think about 'mental health' and in how we try to help people in distress.

## Invalid diagnoses

A medical approach naturally relies on diagnosis. I shall expand on this issue in Chapter 2, but there is precious little science in psychiatric diagnosis. I chose to work in the mental health system anticipating that I would be part of a vital and life-saving system of committed and caring professionals, eager to understand their clients' lives. Over more than twenty years as an active clinician and researcher, I am reluctantly coming to the conclusion, shared by many of my colleagues, that the dominant diagnostic framework in mental health is unreliable, invalid and inhumane and even bizarre. Committees of experts (with clear financial as well as professional advantage in coming to a consensus that supports a 'disease model' in the face of scientific evidence) fail to agree on diagnostic criteria. Statistical analyses fail to identify clusters of symptoms that correspond to the putative 'disorders'. In fact, the abject failure of diagnostic approaches has led the enormously wealthy and enormously influential US NIMH (National Institute of Mental Health) to declare that its strategy 'cannot succeed' if it uses the diagnostic categories enshrined in the influential 'Diagnostic and Statistical Manual' of the American Psychiatric Association (which I shall describe in more detail in Chapter 2), and henceforth will 'be re-orient its research away from [those] categories'.[26] And, as I shall detail in Chapter 2, there is widespread opposition from a wide group of professional and service user-led groups.

Despite this, in the current (flawed) system, diagnostic labels have huge implications – they affect access to healthcare (but they shouldn't), they affect legal issues (but they shouldn't), they affect employment rights (but they shouldn't) and they lead to discrimination and stigma. They are hugely 'sticky'; like zombies, they may well be dead, but they don't realise it and carry on walking. Fortunately, again, however, alternatives are available. A combination of simple problem identification and psychological formulations would address people's problems. As I explain in Chapter 2, a simple list of problems would permit sensible and appropriate planning, and would result in much higher levels of reliability. Validity, too, would be significantly improved, as invalidity in psychiatric diagnosis stems not from the identification of specific problems – whether 'symptoms' (effectively, ways of thinking and acting) or environmental stresses – but from the complex rules for combining these to form diagnoses and the meaning of those diagnoses as representing 'real illnesses'.

## The drugs don't work

Not surprisingly (since the diagnoses don't match onto any patterns of problems we recognise in the real world, and don't relate to any 'biomarkers' – indicators of underlying biological abnormalities), the drugs don't really work, as I'll discuss in more detail in Chapter 3. It's not surprising that pharmaceutical chemicals can affect our mood; the vast majority of us regularly buy mind-altering chemicals every day. Coffee, tea, alcohol and nicotine show both that chemicals can affect our thoughts, moods and behaviour, and that these can have effects (both good and bad) without necessarily treating any illnesses.

Although there are over 47 million prescriptions per year for antidepressant medication in the UK alone, there's plenty of evidence that antidepressants are much less effective than we would like. As I'll explain in more detail in Chapter 3, careful research comparing the long-term outcomes for people taking antidepressant medication with people taking placebos suggests only at best a very marginal benefit.

The same applies to long-term so-called 'anti-psychotic' medication. These drugs often have serious, life-changing (and occasional very noticeable) adverse effects. Because they affect various physical systems, such as our heart, liver and kidneys, as well as our brains, and because one of the common adverse effects is a significant gain in weight (which is, of course, very harmful), these drugs can significantly affect one's health.[27] Outcomes for patients suffering from 'schizophrenia' have not improved since the Victorian age and an increasing number of people are disabled by mental health problems. This contrasts with what has happened in physical medicine, where genuine advances have led to improved outcomes and reduced disability.[28] There is evidence that some forms of pharmacological medication may be helpful in the short term (this is discussed in depth in Joanna Moncrieff's books).[29] But this is, first of all, unsurprising – drugs that act on the brain are not new in human history, and we are well aware of their effects on mood and behaviour. It is also important to note that these effects are not 'cures' (and are even probably not 'treatments') and can have significant negative effects in the longer term. And all this is without mentioning ECT (electroconvulsive therapy).

## Coercion

Mental health care is unusual within healthcare specialities in the use of coercion. Whilst the usual argument goes that coercion is necessary because people 'lack insight', my experience suggests that the main reason is different. While there is a great deal of demand for care, the 'care' and 'treatment' on offer is often not what people want or need. Indeed it can be aversive to the extent that we need to coerce people into accepting it. At any one time, nearly 20,000 people are being detained in psychiatric hospitals against their will, 'sectioned' under the Mental Health Act. These are not just extreme or rare cases, people with a wide range of problems can find themselves caught up in coercive practices.[30] The history of mental health care is an unfortunate history of coercion, with many mental health treatments clearly rooted in moral judgements and punitive approaches.[31] Today, in the context of a general disquiet about a perceived lack of compassion in healthcare, the extent and nature of coercion in mental health care is a clear cause for concern.

Some form of mental health legislation may well be needed, as some people's low mood, risk of suicide, confusion or disturbed behaviour puts them at extreme risk or, in very unusual cases, renders them a risk to others. I contributed to the drafting of both the Mental Health Act and the Mental Capacity Act. It is important to legislate for people whose difficulties put them at significant personal risk, or who pose a risk to others. But this is a social and psychological problem, not a medical one. Diagnosis and even severity of an 'illness' do not relate to risk and dangerousness. Decisions do need to be made about the necessary care of people with serious problems who are at risk. And, after the fact, decisions need to be made about how to deal with people who have committed crimes. In both cases, current practice in a 'disease model' driven system is flawed. A more coherent and fair approach would be to agree to take decisions on behalf of other people if they are unable to make decisions for themselves, regardless of whether they have a diagnosis... and to make judicial decisions in the criminal justice field on the same basis. This doesn't mean 'letting them off'; it means making appropriate decisions on rational bases.

## Psychiatry in crisis and schism

Psychiatry is itself in crisis. As outlined in the major Department of Health report into the status and future of psychiatry ('*New Ways of Working*', in which I was a major participant)[32] rates of divorce, alcohol and drug use, sickness absence and even suicide are higher in psychiatrists than in the general public or other medical specialities. At the same time, recruitment into psychiatry is also in crisis – psychiatry is one of the least popular medical specialities, and consequently the quality of recruits into psychiatry generally tends to be low. Psychiatry is also under fire from outside. Instead of forming groups with names like '...Friends of ...', former patients describe themselves as 'survivors', and they frequently explicitly regard themselves as having survived psychiatry itself rather than being survivors of the distressing experiences for which they sought help.

The discussion of alternative models for the delivery of mental health care is absolutely not a dispute between psychologists and psychiatrists. Sadly, many psychologists themselves use diagnostic labels and, publicly at least, do not question the 'disease model' or the widespread use of psychiatric medication. (Privately, I sometimes wonder whether their beliefs are at least partly influenced by the financial consequences of their practice and our traditional reluctance as a profession to challenge the presently dominant world-view). Equally, many psychiatrists reject these views. Historically, psychiatrists such as R.D. Laing and Jacques Lacan as well as the arch anti-psychiatrist Thomas Szasz all rejected the biomedical, diagnose–treat, model of psychiatry. More recently, a total of 29 eminent psychiatrists co-authored a paper entitled 'Psychiatry beyond the current paradigm',[33] arguing that '...psychiatry needs to move beyond the dominance of the current, technological, paradigm...'.

There is a big difference, then, between what I regard as entirely justifiable scientific scepticism, frustration, sadness, even anger at unscientific, unhelpful, old-fashioned biomedical determinism, disease-model thinking and a diagnose–treat model on the one hand, and scorn for the profession of psychiatry on the other. I have great respect for my colleagues who are psychiatrists, and feel I have learned greatly from those clinical leaders with whom I've worked. As will be made clear throughout this book, my vision for the future of mental health care is predicated on a central role for psychiatry and for psychiatrists. I am opposed to ways of thinking, of service organisations and modes of practice that I believe to be profoundly unhelpful but that doesn't mean I am critical of psychiatrists. This means I need (as I've learned over the years) to distinguish carefully between criticisms of the current ethos and practice of mental health care and criticisms of psychiatry. This occasionally leads to clumsy language – for which I apologise. I shall try to use the phrase 'mental health care' rather than 'psychiatry'. And if, in my frustration, I tar all my psychiatrist colleagues with a biomedical brush, I also apologise.

This crisis is also revealed in internal schism. In the past few years we have seen three very different visions for the future of the profession – from within the profession. The psychiatrist Professor Nick Craddock, in an editorial in the British Journal of Psychiatry, argued that psychiatry needs to re-establish itself as a branch of medicine, re-establish mental ill-health as a medical concept, re-establish the biological and neurological basis of 'real' mental illness and re-establish the authority and status of the psychiatric, medical consultant.[34] Professor Craddock suggested that much of the business of psychiatry is – as I would argue – normal human emotional response to difficult social circumstances. But he suggested that this should be separated from the 'genuine' mental illnesses – leaving the profession of psychiatry in what he would regard as appropriate hierarchical authority in a disease model, medical model, mental health care service. It seems (reading somewhat between the lines of Craddock's article) that he is suggesting that psychiatry should have little to do with 'normal' responses, although this presupposes (wrongly in my opinion) that this is a valid distinction. Pat Bracken, another psychiatrist, and also in an editorial in the British Journal of Psychiatry, argued almost exactly the opposite. He suggested that the vast majority of mental health problems, including those traditionally seen as symptoms of serious 'illnesses' such as 'schizophrenia' should instead be understood from the perspective of social psychiatry – as normal, human, responses to difficult social circumstances. He argued for a social, psychosocial, empathic response. Refreshingly, and rather wonderfully, this stance has been repeated by Dinesh Bhugra, as incoming president of the World Psychiatric Association.[35] Not that different from my own position ... except that Pat Bracken, Dinesh Bhugra and colleagues also argued that this psychosocial perspective was the proper role for psychiatry in a mental health care system still centred on medical primacy. Personally, I would argue that the logical consequence is that, therefore, a medical subspecialty (psychiatry) should play an important contributory role in a predominantly psychosocial service.

A third model emerged from the multi-professional discussions that were part of the 'New Ways of Working' project,[36] championed by the consultant psychiatrist Christine Vize. This model suggested that proper care for people in deep personal distress was a team effort: a multi-professional effort. Since people have a range of needs, from social, through psychological to medical needs (and in different proportions for different people), the team requires a range of specialists who would work together (in different cases in different ways) to offer help. In this model, psychiatry would be a valuable partner, but would have an entirely different – more 'democratic' and much more along the lines of genuine consultancy, contributing to a multidisciplinary mental health care team's work where necessary, rather than necessarily having hegemonic authority.

I strongly orientate to the third model in practice, but have a lot of sympathy with Bracken's approach in terms of ethos and framework of understanding. Rather unexpectedly, I also think that Craddock's approach has merit. In my clinical experience, I have frequently been disappointed at the medical care offered to clients. I am unconvinced that clients are offered the physical healthcare that they need and which is particularly important for people who are both often poor and taking powerful medication. In particular, I think it would be ideal if all clients were able to consult with an expert psychiatrist who was able to understand and explain the mode of action of the medication and its potential risks. I do not always find this expertise in practice. I agree with Nick Craddock that expert medical input should be part of every mental health team. What I do not agree with is that this expertise renders a medical colleague the natural leader of a clinical team, or that a medical perspective is a natural guiding ethos for the service. I therefore conclude that none of these models fully addresses the depth of psychiatry's malaise, and none has a fully-developed solution.

## A psychological ethos and model

We need to develop and implement a new approach to understanding mental health problems. As I outlined in 'New Laws of Psychology',[37] a psychological approach offers a coherent alternative. Our social circumstances, and our biology, influence our emotions, thoughts and behaviours – our mental health – through their effects on psychological processes. This psychological model of mental health and well-being proposes that our biology and our life circumstances both exert their influence through their effect on psychological processes. Of course, all mental health problems involve the brain, for the simple reason that all thoughts we ever have involve the neurological functioning of the brain. But that's not an explanation, merely a more detailed description (it's like explaining warfare in terms of muscular contractions in the fingers on the triggers). In statistical terms, variance in neurological processes seems to account for very little in terms of mental health – or indeed human behaviour in general. Most of the variability in people's problems appears to be explicable in terms of their experience rather than genetic or neurological malfunctions. Neurotransmitters such as serotonin and dopamine are associated with a variety of emotional problems. That's hugely unsurprising; reward mechanisms involve serotonin and dopamine... but that's true for everyone.

Since the 1950s psychologists (and psychiatrists who understand cognitive psychology) have developed sophisticated and practically useful models of how people understand the world. In straightforward terms, people are born as natural learning engines, with highly complex but very receptive brains, ready to understand and then engage with the world. As a consequence of the events we experience in life, we develop mental models of the world, including the social world. We then use these mental models to guide our thoughts, emotions and behaviours.

Understanding things this way suggests that notions such as 'mental illness' and 'abnormal psychology' are old-fashioned, invalid and demeaning, that diagnostic categories such as 'depression' and 'schizophrenia' are unhelpful, and that the concept of mental illness is relatively meaningless. I am certainly not arguing that people are not distressed or that psychological problems do not exist. Many people clearly experience severe psychological distress. As I said above, in the UK, suicide is the most common cause of death in women in the year after the birth of their first child. We all have emotional problems from time to time, and there is a well-recognised statistic that one in four of us will, at some point in our lives, have difficulties severe enough to meet the criteria for a 'mental disorder'. The cost to the state from mental ill-health is estimated at over £100 billion per year, and antidepressant drugs are among the most common – and most profitable – products of the major multinational pharmaceutical companies. But ideas of disease or illness are unhelpful. Even the concept of 'abnormal' psychology is unreasonable: we don't talk about 'abnormal chemistry 'or 'abnormal physics' – the same principles apply whatever value we ascribe to their effects. Instead, we know a lot about the key psychological and developmental processes that make us human, and we know how events in our lives, social circumstances and our biological make-up can affect those processes. Addressing well-being from that perspective is simultaneously radical and common-sense. Scientific research into the psychological processes we all use to understand the world and interact with other people offers a scientifically valid and more helpful approach than the idea of 'mental illnesses'. I will reinforce the World Health Organization's definition of health (that health is more than the absence of illness) and suggest that, rather than researching so-called mental illnesses, we should acknowledge that the concept of mental illness is probably misleading and unhelpful in the first place. Rather, an evidence-based approach to mental well-being – developing and applying our scientific understanding of the key psychological processes that underpin our humanity – offers great hope.

Like Pat Bracken, I believe that human distress is largely a social phenomenon... but I therefore conclude that the role of the psychiatrists within mental health services needs radically to change. In essence, we need to see psychiatry adopt an approach that is both more modest and more democratic. Like Nick Craddock, I believe that psychiatrists have very real and valuable specialist knowledge and skills... and that these should be available to the democratic, team-based, multi-disciplinary services envisioned by Christine Vize. This approach would reverse the current dominance of psychiatric modes of thinking – the 'disease model' and the 'diagnose–treat' model – and place psychiatry in a more appropriate relationship with social and psychological models of care. Although such a change would be challenging both for psychiatrists and for psychologists (who would then be expected both to shoulder the burden of responsibility and to acknowledge the importance of social as well as psychological factors) it is worth spelling out – in detail – the practical consequences of such an approach.

The difficulties that are traditionally thought of as 'mental health' issues are in truth primarily social and psychological problems. Of course, there are physical, biological aspects to them. That's true for all human experiences. But we need to understand that we're trying to respond to social and psychological problems, not treating diseases. And we therefore need a profound change in how we try to help people. We need to move away from a state of affairs where the default response to distress is medical care, whether in the community or in hospital. We need to stop diagnosing 'mental illnesses' and we need to stop prescribing drug treatments. Instead, we need to offer social and psychological interventions. Happily, these can be very effective. Even when people need residential care for very serious crises, there is no reason that this needs to be in hospital; non-medical residential crisis centres which provide social care and support are likely to be much more helpful. That means that a formal transfer of responsibilities of mental health care to local authorities (as has recently happened with public health and is very common across Europe, with a strong tradition of city governance) would be appropriate. This would represent a return to an approach which was common in the past, before distress began to be medicalised in the 19th and 20th centuries. But all that would mean profound changes for the professions of psychiatry and nursing in particular. It would be financially affordable for the nation, but might be challenging for powerful and well-paid professionals. However, the bitter pill I'm prescribing is necessary to cure the grievous sickness of the current system.

Services planned on the basis of a psychosocial model, would offer a very radical alternative. Instead of seeing care for people with mental health problems as a specialist branch of medicine, with links to social care, we would see such support as essentially part of *social provision*, with specialist input from our medical colleagues. In such a world, people would default to a *psychosocial explanatory model*, and the disease model of mental disorder would be redundant. That would, at least in my opinion (but substantiated by considerable evidence) lead to more *empathy*, more *compassion*, more *understanding* of people's needs both by professionals and in wider society, and put a stop to stripping people of their sense of *agency* – their ability to help themselves. People's problems would be understood as just that – problems, and diagnoses would be largely replaced by *formulations*. For people in extreme distress, *places of safety* would still be needed to replace the niche filled at present by in-patient wards. However these should be seen as places of safety, not medical treatment units, should therefore be led by social workers, or possibly psychologists, rather than doctors or nurses, and physically designed as homely, welcoming houses rather than 'wards'. On those units, our medical, psychiatric colleagues would still play a valuable role, but would act as consultants *to* the care team on specifically medical issues, not necessarily leaders *of* those teams. The ethos of care on such units would be based on *recovery*, not treatment or cure, and be firmly based on a psychosocial formulation of the problems facing each service user. Good quality, humane, care, and taking seriously the person's own views about their difficulties and needs rather than insisting that they see themselves as 'ill' and accept medication, would minimise the need for compulsion. When compulsion is needed, however, the legal criteria should be based on the principle that people should only be subject to coercion when they are unable to make the relevant decisions for themselves – a *capacity-based* approach.

For the majority of us, though, mental health care is already community based. In the vision of care proposed here, reconfiguring services as psychosocial rather than medical would transform care. Links to other community-based services such as primary care (GP) and public health services are strong and should remain so. Interestingly, public health services are already based in local authorities. As with in-patient care, medical psychiatrists would be valued to consultants to community mental health teams rather than necessarily leading them. Their ethos would shift from a medical to a psychosocial one, and shift from medical dominance to a model whereby medical colleagues offer consultancy on primarily medical issues (for example the prescription of drugs) to those psychosocial teams.

There should be a very significantly reduced emphasis on drugs. In particular, long-term drug use should be avoided. Where medication is used (sparingly, and short term) it is important that high-quality (and that emphasis is important) medical and pharmaceutical advice is available. Most especially, we must see a significant increase in the range, quality and availability of a wide range of psychosocial interventions – both practical help and psychological therapies. However, the emphasis should be on care and support rather than 'treatment'. This is obviously true in community settings – where it is frankly appalling that people seeking help for social and personal issues are diagnosed with illnesses and given drugs – but is also true in residential settings. In episodes of acute distress, a few people would benefit from very short-term prescription for medication (mainly to help them feel calmer if they are deeply distressed and agitated, or to help them through the depths of despair and 'depression') but three key points follow. First, such use of medication should (following the advice of Jo Moncrieff) be very brief, targeted and practical. Second, following from that, medication should be used to help people through difficult times, not to 'treat' putative 'illnesses'. And finally... there are very real effective alternatives to medication. Many problems resolve from crisis-point to a more manageable state if people are simply offered high quality, genuine care and support. Psychological therapies such as cognitive behavioural therapy (CBT) can be effective for very many people with a wide range of problems, even when those are serious. And non-medical whole-service alternatives such as the Soteria approach[38] appear extremely effective.

**A prescription for mental health and well-being**

Drawing this all together, my prescription for our mental health and well-being services could be summarised as:

1. *Get the message right.* The first step towards a humane, scientific, approach to mental health and well-being is to ensure that we get the message right. We need to change our whole framework of under-standing from a 'disease model' to a 'psychosocial model'. I shall explain this more in the next chapter.
2. *Drop the language of disorder.* We must stop regarding people's very real emotional distress as merely symptoms of diagnosable 'illnesses'. A simple list of people's problems (properly defined) would have greater scientific validity and would be a better basis both for indi-vidual care planning and for the design and planning of services. Again, I will explain more below.
3. *Be careful with medication.* We should sharply reduce our reliance on medication to address emotional distress. Medication should be used sparingly and on the basis of what is needed in a particular situa-tion – for example to help someone sleep or to help someone feel calmer. It should rarely be used long term, and we should not look to medication to 'cure' non-existent underlying 'illnesses'. In practice, this means adopting Dr Joanna Moncrieff's 'drug-based' approach in contrast to the more common 'disease-based' approach.
4. *Offer holistic psychosocial services.* Services should be equipped to address the full range of people's social, personal and psychological needs and also address prevention. Where individual therapy is needed, effective, formulation-based, psychological therapies should be available to all. That means involving a wide range of community workers and psychologists in multidisciplinary teams, and promoting psychosocial rather than medical solutions. All such therapies should be evidence-based and delivered by qualified, competent profes-sionals. Decisions about what therapy or therapies should be offered to whom should be based on a person's specific problems and on the best evidence for the effectiveness of the intervention, not on diag-nosis, and individual formulations should be used to put together an

individualised package of care suitable for addressing each person's unique set of problems. Using psychological therapies as part of a psychosocial, rather than biomedical, approach would significantly change the way clinical psychologists and others work, particularly psychiatrists. Working within a psychosocial ethos, supporting well-being and recovery rather than treating illnesses, is a perfectly respectable medical role for our psychiatric colleagues – exemplified in the roles of those such as general practitioners and public health physicians, and the role of professional medical advisors to athletes.

5. *Offer non-medical residential care.* When people are in crisis, residential care may be needed, but this should not be seen as a medical issue. Since a 'disease-model' is inappropriate, it is also inappropriate to care for people in hospital wards; a different model of care is needed. Residential units should be based on a social, rather than a medical, model. Residential social workers may well be the most appropriate people to be in charge of such units. The nature of extreme distress means that medical colleagues may well be valuable members of the team but again they should be consultants *to* the unit, rather than in charge of the ward. It is likely that the power of the Mental Health Act to detain someone against their will would be needed much less frequently in such a system. Where their use is being considered the decisions we take should be based on the risks that individuals pose to themselves and others, together with their capacity to make decisions about their own care, rather than on whether they have a 'diagnosis'. This approach is already the basis for the law in Scotland. The law in England and Wales allows for the professional who is legally responsible for a person's care – known as the 'responsible clinician' – to be a psychologist, nurse, or social worker. This should be routine. When we abandon a 'disease model' of care and adopt a more humane psychosocial approach, the law relating to mental health could change significantly, with new roles for new professions, and a greater focus on social justice and judicial oversight.

6. *Establish democratic multidisciplinary teams.* Teams should be multidisciplinary, democratic and take a psychosocial approach as their starting point. In the multidisciplinary teams delivering these services, psychiatric colleagues should remain valuable colleagues. An ideal model for interdisciplinary working would see leadership of such teams determined by the skills and personal qualities of the individual members of the team. Our medical colleagues would be consultants *to* the team, not leaders *of* the team.

And so...

7. *Plan for mental health and well-being alongside other social, rather than medical, services.* Mental health services should be based in local authorities, alongside other social, community-based services. That doesn't mean creating teams of doctors and nurses managed out of hospital-based NHS trusts but in a building away from the hospital site. It means that we should locate the whole service in the community – put the service entirely under local authority control. In the UK, we have the model of public health (recently transferred to local authority control) to build upon. Services would then be under democratic local governance. I recognise that some local authorities – especially, perhaps, in developing countries, may not yet be robust enough for the task, but this should be the vision and aspiration, rather than aiming for a medical model.

Adopting this approach would result in much lower reliance on medical interventions, and a much greater reliance on social and psychological forms of help. We would – we may as well be honest – need fewer psychiatrists. As we see a move towards community-based social services, we could look to primary care (general practice – GP) colleagues for much of the necessary medical consultation and input; linking psychological care to the wider well-being of patients in the community. We would, in contrast, require much greater emphasis on, training in, and staffing of, psychosocial approaches. What I'm proposing would be a very major revolution in mental health services and in psychiatric practice.

# 1
# Get the Message Right: A Psychosocial Model of Mental Health and Well-being

*The first step towards a humane, scientific, approach to care is to ensure that we get the message right – we need to change the framework of understanding from a 'disease model' to a 'psychosocial model'. That means recognising that our mental health and well-being depends on the things happen to us, how we make sense of those events and how we respond to them. Differences between people are largely the result of social and psychological influences, rather than reflecting individual pathologies, medical or biological factors. Adopting this approach would be entirely compatible with the best traditions of psychiatry, and may even be the profession's last chance to secure its future.*

Psychiatry is a specialty within medicine, and medical thinking shapes many people's understanding of the nature and causes of psychological distress, and of what constitutes appropriate care. We talk of being 'ill', of taking 'sick leave' from work, of retiring 'on ill-health grounds', of 'diagnosis' and of 'treatment'. Diagnostic manuals are based on the assumption that distress can be diagnosed like any other, physical, illness. Researchers study the 'aetiology', or causation, of problems that are assumed to be illnesses 'like any other'. We have become so used to thinking of psychological distress as a branch of medicine that we are in danger of no longer really challenging this assumption. But we need to start thinking differently. Real positive progress may only be possible when we realise that we are discussing a psychological and social phenomenon, not a medical one.

## Reform and humanity

Textbooks of psychiatry like to present the history of the discipline as a humane progression from superstition and error through to scientific enlightenment. The 18th and 19th centuries saw the care of the 'insane' transferred from the responsibility of local parishes and city authorities to physicians (later alienists and psychiatrists). This is generally accepted to have led to more humane treatment and enlightened care – with Philippe Pinel's work at the 'Pitié-Salpêtrière Hospital' in Paris leading the way. Quite naturally, with the medical profession having responsibility for care, a medical ethos now prevailed. And, as Richard Bentall described in his book 'Madness Explained',[1] leading psychiatrists of the 19th century quite understandably incorporated the latest medical science into their care. So psychiatric diagnosis took hold and biomedical explanations became popular, attempting to emulate the success of similar, hugely important, developments in physical medicine.

It is very tempting to see a causal link between the undoubted progress towards humanity and the medicalisation of our understanding of psychological distress. The two developments happened at the same time, but a more humane approach towards people in distress was not dependent on developments of scientific medicine. Over a couple of hundred years, we saw the care of the 'insane' become the responsibility of physicians, psychiatry incorporated into medicine and simultaneously, significant improvements in the living conditions of many of the previous inmates. However… contrary to the implicit messages offered by many, I am not at all sure that the first development was the cause of the second. So, while Pinel revolutionised care at the Parisian Pitié-Salpêtrière Hospital, in the UK we celebrate the humanity of William Tuke's 'York Retreat', which was conceived of as a social, rather than a medical, initiative (and derided by the establishment of the time). The 18th and 19th centuries saw immense, revolutionary change in a swathe of social systems. Leaving aside the political revolutions of various kinds, both violent and non-violent, that swept across Europe, the past 250 years have seen reform ushering in humane care in many areas. We made impressive strides towards abolishing slavery. In the legal system, we have seen repeal of unjust laws and the development of a range of protection for defendants as well as wholesale reform of jails and regimes of punishment. We have seen the democratic enfranchising of working men and finally women, whereas political participation used to be a privilege for aristocrats and landowners. We have seen the spread of social welfare and (although we're still waiting for the USA to catch up) the development of universal healthcare. Although each of these reforms depended on developments in our scientific and academic understanding of human nature, they did not require a 'medical model'. Change, humane change, is clearly possible without labelling the subject matter as an 'illness'. We can decide to give working men and women a vote without diagnosing the illness of 'disenfranchisement'. We can offer people a decent quality of life if unemployed or retired without diagnosing an illness of 'poverty syndrome'. And we can treat defendants in criminal proceedings with justice and humanity without necessarily invoking illness. Indeed, a churlish commentator may well point out that individual members of the medical profession have occasionally applied a medical approach to oppose rather than promote reform. In 1851, a Dr Samuel A. Cartwright proposed that the pseudo-diagnosis of 'drapetomania' could be used to label the supposed mental illness that caused black slaves to flee captivity. In 1946, the British Medical Association initially opposed the development of the National Health Service, primarily because it was feared it could affect their incomes as private medical practitioners.

This is significant. Enlightened, humane, progressive social services are possible without invoking a medical framework. This is not to deny or minimise the heroic work that pioneering doctors undertook in recent centuries to rescue people from horrendous 'care'. Radical progress was needed, and physicians often led the way. But we do need to question whether a biomedical perspective is now an appropriate way to understand mental health and well-being. And dubious appeals to history are not necessarily useful guides to addressing that issue.

## Debates and disagreements

Discussions about mental health and psychological well-being often unquestioningly assume that the 'disease model' is the only approach. But this assumption is hotly contested, and passionate debates about the essential nature of psychological distress take place even within psychiatry itself. At one end of the spectrum, many authoritative writers have argued that our psychological well-being can largely be explained in terms of brain functioning. This argument is intimately connected to the idea that problems in brain functioning can be diagnosed as 'mental illnesses', explained in biomedical terms, and treated using medical interventions. The 'disease-model' approach to psychiatry is dependent on a biomedical, reductionist view of human nature. Within modern psychiatry, there are many contrasting perspectives.

### Perspective 1 ... 'psychiatry is a medical speciality ... '

It is abundantly clear that many (but not all, by any means) psychiatrists have always been strong proponents of both a biological explanation for mental health problems, and a biological perspective on human behaviour more generally. In 1989, the American Psychiatrist Samuel Guze published a short paper entitled 'Biological psychiatry: is there any other kind?'[2] in which he argued that, since all thoughts, all behaviours and all emotions have their origins in the brain, it is to the physical functioning of the brain that we should look for explanations and ideas for interventions. This general principle was developed by Eric Kandel in his well-written and very influential 1998 article; 'A new intellectual framework for psychiatry'.[3] For Guze and Kandel, changes in biological functioning are the 'final common pathway' for mental disorder and, indeed, therapy. For Kandel and Guze, all the important factors that affect our mental health do so by causing changes in biological functioning. That includes therapy; if therapy works (Guze and Kandel argue), it works by changing the biology of our brains.

More recently, in 2008, Professor Nick Craddock and 36 colleagues from the UK published an unabashed manifesto for the future of psychiatry – entitled 'a wake-up call for British psychiatry'.[4] After acknowledging that improved 'psychosocial care ... is both understandable and welcome', Craddock and colleagues argue that this has been accompanied by the 'creeping devaluation of medicine' in psychiatry. Their argument is that political forces and 'the collusion, or at least the acquiescence, of psychiatrists' has undermined a quintessentially medical approach to psychiatry. They argue that this 'disadvantages patients and is very damaging to both the standing and the understanding of psychiatry in the minds of the public, fellow professionals and ... medical students'.

Craddock and colleagues' perspective is clear. They state: 'British psychiatry faces an identity crisis. A major contributory factor has been the recent trend to downgrade the importance of the core aspects of medical care. In many instances this has resulted in services that are better suited to delivering non-specific psychosocial support rather than a process of thorough, broad-based diagnostic assessment with formulation of aetiology, diagnosis and prognosis followed by specific treatments.' They continue: ' ... Psychiatry is a medical specialty. We believe that psychiatry should behave like other medical specialties.' This is a precise recapitulation of a medical model of psychiatry. Craddock and colleagues are also refreshingly clear in their professional or political aspirations – this is a precise recapitulation of a medical model of psychiatry.

Unlike Guze and Kandel, Craddock and colleagues advance only implicit, not explicit, arguments about biological aetiology. But those implicit references are clear. They take issue with 'the scepticism of some psychiatrists towards biomedical explanations of illness' and argue that there is '…a very real risk that as the understanding of complex human diseases steadily increases, recent moves away from biomedical approaches to psychiatric illness will further marginalise patients….' Most tellingly, Craddock and colleagues argue that: 'Major advances in molecular biology and neuroscience over recent years have provided psychiatry with powerful tools that help to delineate the biological systems involved in psychopathology and impairments suffered by patients. We can be optimistic that over the coming years these advances will facilitate the development of diagnostic approaches with improved biological validity and enhanced clinical utility in terms of predicting treatment response. We can expect that completely novel treatments will be developed based on detailed understanding of pathogenesis.'

In other words, Craddock and colleagues suggest that it is risky to be sceptical about biomedical explanations, that moving away from a biomedical approach would harm patients. They confidently expect that molecular biology and neuroscience will help us understand the 'pathogenesis' (the cause or origin of a disease) of mental health problems, confirm the value of 'biomedical explanations of illness' and reinforce the value of a medical psychiatric profession.

### Perspective 2 … 'psychiatry is not a medical speciality…'

But that is not the only voice from within the profession and academic discipline of psychiatry. Like Nick Craddock, Pat Bracken is also a consultant psychiatrist and professor of psychiatry. He, like Craddock, was able to convene an impressive collection of like-minded psychiatrists and, like Craddock, set out their opinions in an editorial in the British Journal of Psychiatry.[5] Which argued almost exactly the opposite. Pat Bracken and colleagues suggested that the vast majority of mental health problems should be understood from the perspective of social psychiatry – as normal, human responses to difficult social circumstances. And therefore Pat and colleagues argued for a social, psychosocial, empathic response.

There is some value in directly contrasting the views of Nick Craddock and colleagues with those of Pat Bracken and colleagues. Craddock and colleagues suggest that '…Psychiatry is a medical specialty. We believe that psychiatry should behave like other medical specialties', whereas Bracken and colleagues argue that 'Psychiatry is not neurology; it is not a medicine of the brain.' Craddock and colleagues warn that it is 'imperative to take action' to address the negative consequences of 'the scepticism of some psychiatrists towards biomedical explanations of illness' whereas Bracken argues that 'good psychiatry involves active engagement with the complex nature of mental health problems [and] a healthy scepticism for biological reductionism....' And Craddock and colleagues are concerned that '... [recent changes have placed insufficient]... weight on medical fundamentals...', whereas Bracken and colleagues counter that '... good practice in psychiatry primarily involves engagement with the non-technical dimensions of our work such as relationships, meanings and values.' To drive the point home: psychiatry is either a branch of biological medicine... or it's not, that scepticism of biological reductionism is either harmful... or necessary, and a focus on the technical aspects of medicine is either fundamental... or a distraction.

### Perspective 3 ... 'we're a team ...'

The groups led by Nick Craddock and Pat Bracken clearly have divergent views about the future of psychiatry. There is a third approach, which emerged from the multi-professional discussions of 'New Ways of Working',[6] and has been championed by the consultant psychiatrist Christine Vize. This team-based approach argued that proper care for people in deep personal distress is a collective effort; a multi-professional effort. Since people have a range of needs, from social, through psychological to medical (and in different proportions for different people), the team requires a range of specialists who would work together (in different cases in different ways) to offer help. In this model, psychiatry would be a valuable partner, but would have an entirely different – more 'democratic' and much more along the lines of genuine consultancy, contributing to a multidisciplinary mental health care team's work where necessary, rather than necessarily having authority over that team.

I can see elements of value in all three models. I strongly orientate to the third model in practice, but share Pat Bracken and colleagues' approach in terms of ethos and framework of understanding. Perhaps surprisingly, I also think that Craddock's appeal for psychiatrists to remember their core role as medical practitioners has some merit. But I do not believe that any of these models fully addresses the depth of psychiatry's crisis as a profession, and none offers a fully developed solution to the failings of our mental health care system. In particular, these three perspectives together suggest that psychiatry, as it is currently constituted, does not have a coherent or valid model of why people are distressed, nor what might help, and could therefore be either largely irrelevant or actively harmful... but yet (because the principals are psychiatrists) must conclude that psychiatry must remain the key and dominant profession. In essence, I would like to see my psychiatric colleagues hold the pride in their medical expertise that Nick Craddock espouses, adopt the ethos of Pat Bracken, and work democratically within teams as envisaged by Christine Vize.

Things are explicit for Nick Craddock and his colleagues, with a clarion call for the authority of psychiatry to follow from their expertise in biological medicine, since the problem is seen as a biological one, and to be reflected in the nature and ethos of services. It is interesting to note how Craddock and colleagues argue that 'psychiatric services may not be best placed to manage the majority of individuals with such mild symptoms, who would be better served by other more general services. It is probably in the best interest of such individuals to avoid medicalising both the terminology and the type of help that they may require or want.' This is fascinating, because it appears to be a recognition of the psychosocial perspective that I argue throughout this book. But the underlying message is rather darker – it suggests that 'other services' can deal with people with 'mild symptoms', but thereby implies that the medical and medicalised approach – the 'disease model' – remains appropriate for people with more serious problems. My argument is different; I argue that the whole system and ethos needs reform, not that the broken system needs to be retained for the most vulnerable.

Things are different for Pat Bracken and colleagues. But I remain slightly cautious. Bracken argues that 'Psychiatry has the potential to offer leadership in this area.' I would never argue with that, but there are subtle echoes of the idea that psychiatrists, as medical consultants, are naturally placed to lead the teams offering care. This echo can be heard in the active embrace of psychiatry for psychological therapies such as cognitive behavioural therapy (CBT). Obviously this is welcome – it is not only good news that practitioners are offering and advocating appropriate solutions, it is actually good news that people are able to understand the findings of psychological science. It also reflects a phenomenon of medicine; it's quite often driven by 'trial and error' approaches. So, if an intervention 'works', then our clinical colleagues embrace it ... as they probably should. But this has meant that psychological approaches have often been incorporated as afterthoughts into rather conventional services. Many psychologists have expressed some concerns that interventions such as CBT are offered as if they are functionally indistinguishable from medication. That is, people are 'diagnosed' with (for instance) 'mild depression', and 'prescribed CBT'. The outcome, it is hoped, is that the 'symptoms' of 'depression' will be ameliorated. There is little functional difference to prescribing Prozac. And many psychologists are somewhat uncomfortable with that. They would – I would – prefer the entire system to change; for people to have their problems understood rather than diagnosed, and appropriate help offered, not treatment prescribed.

And this argument extends a little, I'm afraid, to the otherwise valuable work of the 'new ways of working' group. I find the conclusions of 'new ways of working', as championed by Christine Vize, very positive, but they have proved controversial among some psychiatrists. Indeed, Nick Craddock takes time to contrast this distributed responsibility model with the vision of him and his colleagues – asking 'if a member of your family were a patient, is a distributed responsibility model the one for which you would opt?' My own answer, of course, is 'absolutely, yes!' As I shall explain later, a multidisciplinary approach is exactly what I would choose, and within such an approach, we give each professional appropriate responsibility. The 'new ways of working initiative' was initiated jointly by the UK's Royal College of Psychiatrists and Department of Health, and had the joint aims of improving care and addressing certain problems within psychiatry – such as its struggle to recruit, and the high levels of stress seen in clinicians. It was, in essence, a plan to help secure and improve the profession. Its conclusion echoed Pat Bracken's views, my views and, in my opinion, the needs of service users. However, it didn't meet the needs of those consultant psychiatrists for whom it seems imperative to remain (in Nick Craddock's words) the 'leader in the clinical team'. Once again, I feel a more fundamental change is needed.

## A new model of mental health and well-being

Many people have called for radical alternatives to traditional models of care. I agree. But I don't think that we need to develop new alternatives. We already have robust and effective alternatives...we just need to use them.

Clinical psychology is a wonderful profession – I'm proud to be a clinical psychologist. But we have, I believe, been tempted down a medical route. We've tended to talk – and sometimes even to think – in terms of 'disorder', in terms of 'aetiology' and in terms of 'pathology' or 'abnormality'. We call our conversations with service users 'therapies' or 'psychological treatments' and conduct 'randomised controlled trials' to test them. We set up programmes such as the UK's 'IAPT' – Improving Access to Psychological Therapies – which is predicated on the notion of identifying people with recognised 'mental disorders', offering 'treatment' and assessing the outcome on the basis of quite traditional medicalised criteria such as the number of 'cases' which 'recover'.[7] We criticise this language, this way of thinking. But all too often, we too use it. We need to place people and human psychology central in our thinking. And we need to return to core principles – ethical, professional and scientific.

The Roman emperor and philosopher, Marcus Aurelius (played by Richard Harris in the film 'Gladiator') once argued that we need always to ask: 'What is this, fundamentally? What is its nature and substance, its reason for being?' What, then, is the fundamental nature and substance of those psychological, emotional and behavioural problems that people label as 'mental health problems'? In my view, they are fundamentally social and psychological issues. They do have clear biological elements – our psychological health is intimately linked to our physical health. So psychologists, therapists and social workers need to work closely along-side GPs, public health physicians and nurses. But mental well-being is fundamentally a psychological and social phenomenon, with medical aspects. It is not, fundamentally, a medical phenomenon with additional psychological and social elements.

The well-established ethos of the clinical psychologist as 'scientist–practitioner' means that we can offer evidence-based scientific models of both mental health problems and well-being. These describe how the social determinants of health and well-being interact with psychological processes. Fundamentally, our thoughts, our emotions, our behaviour and therefore our mental health, are largely dependent on our under-standing of the world, our thoughts about ourselves, other people, the future, and the world. This understanding, of course, has itself been and continues to be shaped by our experiences. Essentially, things happen to us, we make sense of those events and respond to them, and there are consequences. We all differ in the ways we respond to events, and there are many reasons for those differences. There are as many different reasons for these different responses as there are people in the world. Biological factors, social factors, circumstantial factors – our learning as human beings – affect us as those external factors impact on the key psychological processes that help us build up our sense of who we are and the way the world works.

And, of course, if psychological mechanisms (the ways we think, feel and react) mediate the effects of our biological makeup, circum-stances, experiences and relationships on our mental well-being, this implies that psychological interventions – which affect these psycho-logical mechanisms – are likely to be helpful. For example, colleagues and I found – in research conducted with the support of the BBC – that negative life events were substantial contributors to a person's levels of depression and anxiety. Importantly, however, the level of distress that people reported was most strongly influenced by the degree to which people dwelt on their problems, or 'ruminated'. In simple terms, if we were able to 'turn off' our rumination, we'd be able to turn down at least some of our depression and anxiety.

## Prevention beyond the 'disease model'

Advances in the psychological understanding of mental health and well-being allow us to foresee a future beyond the 'disease model'. First, it's important to address the root causes of distress. The ethos of mental health that I'd like to see does place the person at the centre of their universe, and emphasises our individual agency, but it does not imply that people (or their thinking) can be blamed for their distress. The way that people make sense of what happens to them plays an important role and is often a useful focus when we are trying to help someone. However, the most powerful determinants of mental health are the events and circumstances of people's lives. If we are to protect people's mental health, we need wider social or even political change. This is often a neglected topic, but social and political changes are likely to make much more difference overall than anything individuals can do alone.

For example, many people diagnosed with 'psychosis' have experienced poverty. Addressing poverty is rightly the cornerstone of government, and few politicians suggest differently (although many of us fear that right-wing governments pay only lip-service to this aspiration, whilst presiding over policies that actually increase inequalities). With a very specific focus on mental health, however, measures to reduce or eliminate poverty, especially childhood poverty, would be hugely beneficial. However absolute income is not the only important issue. Evidence shows that a major contribution to serious emotional distress is income inequality – the growing gap between the richest and poorest people in society. In their book 'The Spirit Level', sociologists Richard Wilkinson and Kate Pickett demonstrate that mental health problems are highest in those countries with the greatest gaps between rich and poor, and lowest in countries with smaller differences.[8] This suggests that an effective way to reduce rates of mental health problems might be to reduce inequality in society.

Experiences of abuse in childhood are also hugely important. Rates of mental health problems would plummet if we found better ways of protecting children from abuse. This means working with teachers, social workers, community nurses, GPs and the police to identify and then respond to early warning signs that children might be exposed to sexual, physical or emotional abuse or neglect. It also means taking a serious look as a society at what we can do to bring down overall rates of abuse. Bullying – that is, peer-on-peer bullying in school and in leisure settings – is also important, and again here teachers and youth leaders could help … and thereby help prevent later mental health problems.

In that context, we also know that experiences of discrimination are important – people who have been subjected to racism, homophobia and sexual discrimination are put at risk by these experiences. Society – and important agents in society – can help. We can help to make societies less discriminatory. On the other side of this equation, we can perhaps think of ways in which community leaders could help make communities more trusting, more open to help one another – more 'prosocial' in psychological jargon.

And finally, many recreational drugs are associated with mental health problems. Alcohol is unquestionably the most serious substance-related public health issue, but cannabis and other more traditional 'drugs' have been associated with mental health problems in general and psychosis in particular. This certainly doesn't mean that we need a stronger clamp-down on drugs – the so-called 'war on drugs' does not appear to have been won, and many people argue that de-criminalising the possession and use of drugs would be an important positive step towards protecting people's health.

To conclude, the most effective way of reducing rates of mental health problems in our country would be to focus on the social causes of distress. This involves all of us, not just mental health professionals. Politicians in particular have a very important role to play in passing legislation that could protect our health, strengthen our community and prevent mental health problems.

So a new ethos for mental health – moving away from the 'disease model' – would embrace social change. But we must also address the issue of biology. Every thought I have involves a brain-based event. All learning involves changes in associative networks, depolarisation thresholds, synaptic biomechanics, even gene expression. My view is not anti-brain or anti-psychiatry. But I believe that my brain is a learning engine – a biological system that is the servant of learning. I am not the slave of my brain, my brain is the organ with which I learn. So of course every thought involves brain-based activity. But this isn't the same as biomedical reductionism. Our biology provides us with a fantastically elegant learning engine. But we learn as a result of the events that happen to us – it's because of our development and our learning as human beings that we see the world in the way that we do.

This approach contrasts with the approach taken by biological psychiatry. I mentioned psychiatrists Eric Kandel and Samuel Guze earlier. They and their colleagues argue that all psychological concepts will disappear from the psychiatric lexicon as we understand the neural basis of behaviour. Their logic is that any changes in our thinking or behaviour – whether that means learning during childhood, the impact of life experiences or even therapy – reflect physical changes in the neural associative networks. So, they argue, when we understand the physical changes that happen in the brain – the changed 'excitation thresholds', the new synapses etc. – we will understand human behaviour. On one level, this analysis is obviously true. Any learning must involve biological changes in the brain at the molecular and synaptic level. But such an argument is intellectually trivial. All learning – all human behaviour – is dependent on the functioning of the brain. But merely invoking 'the brain' doesn't explain the learning satisfactorily, at least not for me. Of course, a well-functioning brain is necessary for all human activities. But it doesn't really explain why I do one thing in one situation (whereas somebody else behaves differently) or why I behave differently in other situations. To understand that, we need to ask whether such differences between people are best explained by differences in their biology.

Everybody recognises that there are changes in our brains that can affect our thinking, our moods and our behaviour. All over the world people use a range of chemicals – cannabis, alcohol, even caffeine – that affect our psychological functioning because of the effects they have on our brain. Individual differences between people, including genetic differences, naturally affect our behaviour and thinking. There's nothing un-psychological and certainly nothing un-scientific about understanding that biological factors can affect our psychological functioning... and thereby affect our moods, our thinking, our behaviour. But I think there's a world of difference between acknowledging these influences and accepting a 'disease model'. For two reasons.

Firstly, I believe that the relative influence of biological factors is comparatively small. To be slightly more precise, my reading of the available literature suggests to me that the influence of biological variance between people has much less influence on their subsequent emotional life than the variance in their social circumstances.

In my department at Liverpool University, colleagues Ben Barr, David Taylor-Robinson, Alex Scott-Samuel, Martin McKee and David Stuckler demonstrated that around 1000 more people killed themselves in the years between 2008 and 2010 than would have been expected. They also found that the English regions with the largest rises in unemployment had the largest increases in suicides, particularly among men. They conclude that the economic recession was the most likely cause.[9] Recession, economic insecurity, losing your job clearly has a major impact. On a different but related note, my colleagues Richard Bentall and John Read have analysed the impact of childhood trauma – abuse – on the likelihood of developing psychosis. In a number of studies, they have concluded that childhood abuse more than doubles the risk that you'll develop hallucinations or delusional beliefs in later life. The social circumstances of our lives are very significant.

There have been relatively few studies directly comparing the relative contributions of biological and social variables. One attempt was made by Steven Reich and colleagues, who found that life events were much more predictive of future depression than a biological variable that scientists had thought might be important, namely differences in genes that affect a brain chemical called serotonin. It's perhaps noteworthy that proponents of biological reductionism occasionally make some peculiar suggestions, such as the response to research by Bentall and Read, referred to earlier, which suggested that genetic abnormalities might make children vulnerable to BOTH abuse and psychosis, but that the abuse wasn't really the cause.[10] And, of course, when serotonin reuptake genes are found to be less clearly related to depression than might be thought, well, the media 'spin' is that new genetic breakthroughs are likely 'within months'.

## Pathways to mental health

We must also remain clear-sighted as to *how* biological, and, for that matter, social and circumstantial factors affect our mental health and well-being. And, again, the alternative to the 'disease model' is already with us. It's already part of our scientist–practitioner model, and already well-established within psychological science. As just one example, in one piece of research that I have been involved in, we used fMRI technology – functional magnetic resonance imaging – to study regional blood flow during a 'self-referential' task. That is, a task in which the research participants were asked to decide whether particular words were good descriptors of their personality. We found that specific areas of the brain were associated with self-referential thinking, and that these areas were more active in people seeking help for depression. So, when we think – in this example – of ourselves, as opposed to thinking of another person, it's abundantly clear that specific neural pathways are involved. Since thought involves neural signals in the brain, it's hugely unsurprising that thoughts of all kinds involve identifiable brain circuitry.

But identifying a pathway to a particular thought process does not imply that a pathological mechanism has been found. In fact, a much simpler explanation is that, if a particular neural pathway is found to be associated both with emotional and interpersonal difficulties and a key psychological process, then this is an important scientific finding that applies to us all, not just those of us unfortunate enough to have somebody attach an 'illness' label to our emotions. This is not a style of thinking compatible with the 'disease model'. Because every thought must involve a neurological process, merely finding a neurological correlate of emotional distress or psychological process isn't the same as identifying a pathology or an 'illness'.

One colleague suggested I was proposing a 'psychobiosoical model'. I quite like that.

## A psychological model

As a practicing clinical psychologist, I'd go slightly further. Although I argue strongly that social circumstances are important, I think that psychological processes play a central role in our mental health.

I have argued for a long time[11] that mental health is an essentially psychological phenomenon, and that biological, social, and circumstantial factors affect our mental health and well-being by disrupting or

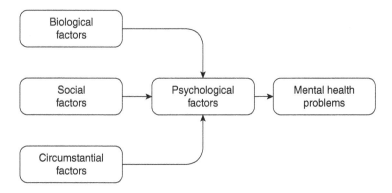

*Figure 1.1*   A psychological model of mental health © Peter Kinderman (2014)

disturbing psychological processes. This places psychology at the heart of mental health.

My work as an academic clinical psychologist has convinced me that how we think, feel and behave – our mental health, in other words – is in large part determined by how we see the world; our thoughts about ourselves, other people, the world and the future. Of course, none of us is free from the influence of nature and nurture, genes and environment. However one important way that they influence us is by shaping how we make sense of the world. Moreover, it seems clear to me that differences between people in how they make sense of the world is best understood in terms of differences in their personal lives, those social, relational and psychological events that have shaped them as human beings. I'm confident that the way we see the world depends more on the experiences we've had in life than on differences in our genes. Either way, it's how we make sense of the world that matters.

Many commentators have pointed out that genetic factors play a role in many mental health problems, and particularly in those problems that can lead to a diagnosis of 'schizophrenia'. More specifically, psychotic phenomena, and particularly hallucinations, have been linked to genetic processes related to differences between people in terms of cerebral lateralization; the degree to which the two hemispheres of the brain are specialised for particular cognitive functions. Several researchers have reported that people who hear voices may have less lateralized cerebral hemispheres, and that this particularly affects the language processing areas. Understandably, genetic factors are believed to be important in this phenomenon.

But to me as a psychologist, auditory hallucinations (voices heard when there is no one there) seem best understood as misattributed cognitions – unspoken (or sometime muttered) and unrecognised thoughts. The key process here is that the thoughts are not recognised by the individual as being internally generated, and instead are attributed to external speakers. The question is then what might lead some people, and not others, to make this attribution. Genetic factors associated with lateralization in the areas of the brain relevant to language processing may well affect 'source monitoring' (the technical term for the ability to tell whether a voice originates internally or externally); so will other biological factors such as taking street drugs or prescribed medication, or being tired or physically unwell. Biological factors obviously affect all decision-making, including deciding whether a voice is real or not, because the mechanism that we use to perform that psychological process is the brain, and the brain is a biological organ. But social or environmental factors can equally impact on our ability to separate different perceptual experiences. Our source monitoring system is influenced by factors such as noise, stress and, crucially, by prior experience of traumatic events, bullying and abuse.

So both biological and environmental factors exert their influence on our mental health by means of their impact on psychological processes. Biological factors have psychological consequences. But so do social and environmental factors. Poverty and social deprivation, and sexual, emotional, or physical abuse can lead to disillusionment, hopelessness, and learned helplessness – to a belief that others are likely to be malevolent, and that there is little or nothing that one can do to improve or change one's lot in life and so there is little point in trying. It should not be surprising if people experiencing such negative events become depressed.

A fully psychological approach to mental health would suggest that our beliefs, emotions and behaviours – including our mental health – are the product of the way we think about the world, our thoughts about ourselves, other people, the world and the future. And it would acknowledge that thoughts are, in turn, the product of a process of learning. Our brain is uniquely efficient at learning, and we actively make sense of our experiences. Our experiences, the life events we've encountered, our social circumstances and, importantly, how we have understood and responded to these experiences, have all shaped our understanding of the world. We need to move beyond the 'disease model' – the idea that emotional problems stem from illnesses which can be diagnosed and treated like any other physical illness. We need to recognise how people have learned to make sense of the world.

## Where would this leave psychiatry?

The model of mental health care I envisage is not greatly different from that proposed by Pat Bracken and his psychiatric colleagues. So there is no inherent or inevitable challenge – this is a model not only compatible with the best traditions of psychiatry (as Pat Bracken and colleagues would see them) but sympathetic to them. Perhaps surprisingly, I also believe this model to be largely compatible with the vision of psychiatry as a valued medical specialism put forward by Nick Craddock and colleagues…when seen through the lens of the 'new ways of working' analysis. I envisage multi-disciplinary mental health care teams offering the holistic care that people need, with democratic and equitable working practices, but following a predominantly psychosocial model. In that vision, there remains a valued place for medical colleagues as they apply their specialist medical knowledge and expertise, as needed.

I would have three caveats, however. First, this perspective sees psychiatric colleagues as consultants to teams, with a specialist and specific role, rather than necessarily offering leadership. This contrasts with Nick Craddock's vision of a dominant biomedical ethos where medical practitioners assume a dominant role in terms of leadership and management as well as in relation to the diagnosis and clinical treatment of 'illnesses'. In the vision I am proposing, medical perspectives are seen as hugely valuable, but as valuable elements of a 'psycho-biosocial' model, not as the inevitable dominant influence. My second caveat is that, therefore, I would expect a proportionate rebalancing of the investment in medical as opposed to psychosocial approaches. Of course, many of my psychiatric colleagues are – as Pat Bracken and colleagues recommend – themselves specialists in psychosocial interventions. Nevertheless, a genuinely psychosocial approach to emotional well-being would need to see a significant investment in the 'psycho' and 'social' aspects of services, and perhaps some rebalancing away from the 'bio' or medical side. Which leads to my third and final caveat. In the future, some thought should be given as to whether GPs (primary care or family doctors) might be the best-placed medical practitioners to offer a medical perspective to the work of community multidisciplinary mental health teams. I recognise that GPs and family doctors are under great pressure in the UK at present. And I recognise that many nations have less well-provisioned primary care medical services. Nevertheless, on first principles, I believe that the most appropriate sub-discipline within medicine to offer this kind of help is the more holistic, more integrative, services of GPs.

So...

The first step towards a humane, scientific, approach to care is to get the message right – to change the framework of understanding from a 'disease model' to a 'psychological model'. This would stress how our 'mental health' depends on the things that happen to us and how we make sense of and respond to those circumstances and events. We all respond in different ways, and there are many reasons for these differences. Our thoughts, our emotions, our behaviour and therefore, our mental health depend on our understanding of the world, our thoughts about ourselves, other people, the future, and the world. There are as many reasons for these different responses as there are people in the world. Biological factors, social factors, circumstantial factors exert their influence through our learning as human beings and their impact on the key psychological processes that help us build up our sense of who we are and the way the world works.

This approach is fundamentally different from a biomedical one. Adopting this approach would be entirely compatible with the best traditions of psychiatry, and would leave psychiatry – especially social psychiatry – as a key profession in a multidisciplinary service. Indeed, adopting such a model may be the profession's best and safest route forwards.

So the first step we need to take towards a humane, scientific, approach to care is to ensure that we get the message right – we need to drop the 'disease model' and adopt a 'psychosocial model'.

# 2
# Understand, Don't Diagnose

*We must stop regarding people's distress as merely the symptom of diagnos-*
*able 'illnesses' and instead develop a more appropriate system for describing*
*and defining people's emotional problems. Traditional psychiatric diag-*
*noses are arbitrary and invalid, and do not map onto biological processes*
*or describe real illnesses. They are also circular concepts, attempting to*
*explain human behaviour merely by labelling it as pathological. This rein-*
*forces a reductionist biological view of mental health and well-being and*
*encourages discrimination and the use of inappropriate medical treatments.*
*Traditional psychiatric diagnoses therefore do more harm than good;*
*instead a simple list of well-defined specific phenomena would be more*
*than sufficient as a basis for individual care planning and for the design*
*and commissioning of services.*

One of the major problems with the 'disease model' of mental health
and well-being is that it relies heavily on diagnosis in order to 'treat'
people's distress. Guided by the flawed assumption that distress is best
thought of as a 'symptom' of an 'illness', mental health professionals go
on to assume that if a set of symptoms has a name, we know what 'it' is,
we can talk to 'patients' about it easily and we have a recognised path of
treatment that will 'cure' it. Unfortunately for this way of thinking about
things, the real world does not appear to want to play along. And, while
medical professionals are naturally inclined to think this way, there are
alternatives.

In his masterpiece 'Billy Budd', left unfinished at his death in 1891
and published in 1924, the American author Herman Melville discusses
the complex relationship between 'sanity' and 'insanity'.

Who in the rainbow can draw the line where the violet tint ends and
the orange tint begins? Distinctly we see the difference of the colors,

but where exactly does the one first blendingly enter into the other? So with sanity and insanity. In pronounced cases there is no question about them. But in some supposed cases, in various degrees supposedly less pronounced, to draw the exact line of demarcation few will undertake tho' for a fee some professional experts will. There is nothing nameable but that some men will undertake to do it for pay.

## A dog chasing its tail

Does giving medical names to distress always help us to understand it? In my opinion, diagnosis is a superficially attractive, but ultimately an inappropriate and unhelpful response. Psychiatric diagnoses convey the idea that people's emotional difficulties can be understood in the same way as bodily diseases. One consequence of this idea is that we fail to look for meaning in people's 'disordered' responses and experiences. It also implies that people need 'expert' help and that their own skills and resources are not enough. Worse still, diagnoses are used as pseudo-explanations for troubling behaviours, for example 'this person is hearing voices because they have schizophrenia'. Many people, perhaps even most people, who hear voices don't find them distressing. But for others they *are* distressing, and these are the people who might seek help from mental health services and receive a diagnosis. Within the disease-model approach, the voices ('hallucinations') are seen as symptoms of 'schizophrenia' – there is a 'mental illness' called 'schizophrenia', and hallucinations are a common 'symptom' of that illness. But, at the same time, the hallucinations are caused by the schizophrenia – 'why is that person hallucinating?', 'because she has schizophrenia', 'how do we know she has schizophrenia?', 'because she's experiencing hallucinations'. It's a circular argument; the dog is chasing its own tail.

   Diagnosis in mental health is a flawed and inappropriate technique. Apart from its circularity, the diagnostic approach fails to appreciate the broader context of a person's experience. Diagnoses take no account of whether a person has had significant losses, has been victimised or abused (whether recently or as a child), or has experienced any other environmental stresses. There are two exceptions, namely diagnoses that do include such information, one explicitly and one implicitly. The diagnosis of 'post traumatic stress disorder' or PTSD is distinctive in that, in order to receive this diagnosis, the person must have experienced a very stressful (traumatic, potentially life-changing) event. There is also a diagnosis of 'adjustment disorder', which can be cynically interpreted as the 'something bad has happened and you've been upset by it...disorder'. These two diagnoses, however, demonstrate the inadequacy of the diagnostic process in this respect. The reference to external, causal factors in both 'PTSD' and 'adjustment disorder' merely highlights how external factors are omitted from all other diagnoses. And this is important. These simple things are profoundly influential. The fact that 'PTSD' is identified as a 'disorder' that represents a response to traumatic external events seems to reinforce the idea that 'depression' or 'personality disorders' are, by contrast, not in any way related to such traumas. This, in turn, means that a person's social and interpersonal difficulties are often ignored in the hope that the right medication regimen will achieve the desired return to normal functioning.

In my experience, the system of psychiatric diagnosis is demeaning and dehumanising. People in distress are not simply a set of symptoms to be assessed and classified. At the point when people most need – and deserve – to be shown empathy and understanding, when they need their individual circumstances to be recognised and taken into account, they are instead merely given a label and allocated to a category within a flawed and out-dated system.

The 'disease-model' approach and its principal tool of diagnosis tend to minimise and ignore issues such as poverty, deprivation, social isolation and childhood abuse. All these experiences lead to distress, and our natural and understandably human responses are then (mis)diagnosed as mental disorders. Giving someone in distress a diagnosis of an 'illness' is essentially futile; merely giving something a name doesn't make it easier for the person to deal with or offer any hope of a solution. We need to lose the labels and start thinking about mental health issues in a different way, with less emphasis on what is 'wrong' with people and more on how and why they feel or act the way they do.

Ultimately, I believe there is no place for medical diagnosis in mental health care. It is at best unhelpful and at worst harmful. At the very least it is an inappropriate and blunt tool to deal with complex psychological events. This is a challenging assumption and one I recognise goes against many decades of accepted wisdom, at least in psychiatric circles (many people in the real world seem to understand these issues rather better). It may sound revolutionary, but I believe that both the history of mental healthcare and scientific research have already proved diagnosis to be problematic and dangerous.

## If we don't learn from history, we are doomed to repeat it

To get an idea of both the problems with diagnosis and how we could live without it, consider the history of how psychiatry has regarded homosexuality. In early versions of psychiatric diagnostic manuals, 'homosexuality' was listed as a mental illness. We have more enlightened ideas now, thankfully. It was while I was writing this book that the World War II code-breaker Alan Turing finally won an official pardon from the UK Government. Turing committed suicide after being prosecuted for an indecency offence – he had been the victim of a theft by his lover and when he reported it to the police, his sexuality was both criminalised and pathologised. Forced to take female sex hormones to emasculate himself, Turing killed himself with a bite from a cyanide-coated apple. If homosexuality were still categorised as a 'mental illness', no doubt we would be seeing frequent publication of academic articles exploring the genetic basis of the 'disorder', its biochemical and neurotransmitter profile and randomised controlled trials of medication designed to 'cure' it. We do see occasional attempts by religiously motivated therapists to this end. But largely, we celebrate peoples' rights to live their lives and express their sexuality as they see fit. We can see life beyond the diagnostic paradigm.

We (or most of us) have learned to view homosexuality as part of a spectrum of sexual identities. So, why can't we see depression, anxiety or paranoia as points on a continuum of normal reactions to distress? People feel and behave differently as a result of trauma, life experiences, upbringing, social status, environment and so on, and often need help to deal with that. Giving these reactions a name – and, consequently, medical 'treatments' – doesn't make living with those human consequences any easier.

So, why are we, as a society, so convinced of the importance of diagnosis?

## People are reassured by diagnoses

Many people actively want their doctor to give a diagnosis. People are dissatisfied when they do not receive a diagnosis and often describe their 'struggles' in obtaining a diagnosis from an unresponsive system. Giving a name to our distress serves a function and, after all, naming something is an important psychological event. If you are plagued by thoughts of being a terrible parent whose children would be better off without you, hearing that you are 'ill' and that what you are experiencing has a name and can be treated, can be very reassuring. You're not going mad, you're not a bad mother, you're not mistaken...you're just ill and can be fixed.

When you look in detail at what medical diagnoses do and don't mean, you might wonder why people find them reassuring. Some of course are hugely valid and important. For example, government campaigns urge us to look out for blood in our bowel movements. This is important, because that can be a symptom of bowel cancer. And, to drive the point home, recognising that you have bowel cancer is something that is not merely synonymous with having blood in the toilet, it is entirely the province of medicine, and the diagnosis (of cancer) is clearly more than the symptom (the blood itself). But in mental health, especially, that logic seems to falter. The 'diagnoses' often appear to be nothing more than a very brief repetition of the problems that the person took to the doctor. This happens occasionally in physical health, too. A person may go to a doctor complaining that their hair is falling out and get told that they have 'alopecia'. They may add that they think the hair has started falling out after a period of considerable emotional stress and be told they have 'stress-related alopecia' or perhaps 'alopecia NOS'. The 'NOS' is shorthand for 'not otherwise specified'. The person has gone to their doctor reporting that their hair is falling out, the doctor has trans-lated that into 'alopecia' and – me included – we feel somehow reassured by this. It's perhaps significant that the diagnoses are often in Latin or Greek. The languages of tradition, of academic authority, of antiquity and of the clerics carry a lot of symbolic weight.

In practice, of course, there is more happening here than merely the diagnosis itself. The diagnosis, the tone of voice, the non-verbal behav-iours and so on all tell the patient that the doctor has heard and, to a degree, understood their problems. The technical, slightly obscure, language, indicates that the doctor is an expert in the field, and conveys confidence. However, despite these potential or possible benefits, a cool and dispassionate look at the data suggests it may be difficult to make valid, reliable or useful diagnoses of psychological problems.

## Getting in the way of empathy

A few years ago, at the University of Liverpool, led by Erika Setzu, we conducted a simple research study into how people understood and explained their mental health problems. We asked people who either had been, or were currently, receiving care in residential psychiatric units, about the circumstances of being admitted to hospital and the ways in which they understood their experiences. One interview went as follows:

> ERIKA: 'Do you know why [the problems began]?'
> INTERVIEWEE: 'No, I don't know for certain. I had taken some pot before my first admission and I thought somebody might have

dropped some acid on it. I also had a difficult childhood. I was physically and emotionally abused, sexually abused as well. This is very difficult for me to get my head round.'

A little later, the interview continued:

> INTERVIEWEE: 'I started to hear voices, but they were not nice voices, they were horrible.'
> ERIKA: 'Did you recognise them?'
> INTERVIEWEE: 'It was the man that abused me…I met this man that was a builder, in construction, you know? And he said that he wanted to give me a job, but they were all lies, he was trying to con me. He took me back to his house, he locked the door and he had sex with me.…And then other voices as well. I went to…hospital and the nurses were very good to me.'
> ERIKA: 'When you went to hospital what did they say it was wrong with you?'
> INTERVIEWEE: 'Schizophrenia, paranoid schizophrenia.'
> ERIKA: 'What do you think personally?'
> INTERVIEWEE: 'What do you mean?'
> ERIKA: 'Do you think it is what you've got?'
> INTERVIEWEE: 'Oh yes, that's what I have got.'[1]

The most important to say is that – despite my criticisms of the 'disease-model' system of care that has evolved – I would criticise nobody involved in this man's care. Indeed, I believe that those caring for him performed their roles admirably. I would, of course, like to see the people who physically, emotionally and sexually abused him arrested and prosecuted. But I think the hospital staff offered him nothing but support and active, positive help. I think that it is appropriate that he approached medical staff for help, as that is (currently at least) the route to obtain help. And I have no doubt that he received proper care. Given the nature of his distress, I suspect that residential care and even (low dose, short-term) medication may well have been helpful. When people have been terribly abused, they can occasionally become so distressed – for example as a result of post-traumatic 'flash-back' memories – that they need this kind of help. If the distress is acute and someone is hearing abusive voices, medication can be a relief. If people need help and a place to stay, at present psychiatric hospitals may be the only realistic option…although, as I shall explain later, I would like to see 'psychiatric wards' replaced with residential units based on a social model. And I can see a role for psychiatric medication, if used appropriately. In fact, medication may well be helpful if it targets those neurological mechanisms that underpin the source-monitoring problems that may contribute to the experience of hallucinations. In summary, I don't think that the nursing and medical professionals treated this man badly.

But I believe it is nonsensical to describe this man's experiences as 'paranoid schizophrenia'. It misses the point. I am confident that the diagnosis in this example was technically accurate – that is, reporting third person auditory hallucinations that cause distress justifies diagnosis of 'paranoid schizophrenia' in standard diagnostic manuals. But it simply fails to identify the man's problems adequately. The label – the diagnosis of 'paranoid schizophrenia' – is unnecessary, it doesn't capture his experiences (neither the experience of hearing voices nor his explanation of the reasons for it) and doesn't distinguish his experiences from other people's. The interviewee reports a childhood history of physical, emotional and sexual abuse, recreational drug use, and traumatic, sexual, assaults in adulthood. In particular, he describes how the adult rapist's voice returned as hallucinations, accompanied by other voices. The label fails to explain the link between the voices and the traumatic events to which they are related. This man's story is entirely understandable on a human level. Not only do we not need this label in order to understand his experiences, but the diagnostic label of 'paranoid schizophrenia' gets in the way. Despite the assumptions of the traditional 'disease model' of diagnostic psychiatry, his story alone has quite a lot of explanatory power, we can quite easily understand this story. The diagnostic label seems redundant after we've heard his story – it seems utterly foolish and inhumane to imply that, in some way, the 'illness' of 'paranoid schizophrenia' has caused these voices. We know – he told us – what led to the voices. 'Paranoid schizophrenia' medicalises, alienates and confuses rather than elucidates. Moreover, it arguably adds to the man's problems by introducing the idea that in addition to his existing misfortunes he also has a brain disease.

Equally, this man's story is unique. Other people, including some of my own friends and relatives, have also been given this label, without any point of similarity in their histories. What they share, what has led people to attach that label to them (the label sticks to them, not to the disembodied 'symptoms'), are certain relatively common experiences such as hearing voices or having crippling fears about other people. As I will explain below, hearing voices is common – very common – while being raped while working as a casual electrician is more specific and, thankfully, rarer. There are hundreds of thousands of people – probably millions of people – who hear voices and many become distressed. Their stories are ALL important and unique. Reductionist diagnoses like 'paranoid schizophrenia' divert attention away from these individual stories and the links between people's lives and their so-called 'symptoms'. And it's worth pointing out that, as well as reductionist, such labels are misleading. To attach the prefix of 'paranoid' to the diagnosis of 'schizophrenia' tends to imply traits of violence, suspiciousness or delusional beliefs, which can further undermine the truth of the stories being told. If a person is 'paranoid' and 'delusional', why bother calling the police about some supposed rapists…?

## Not everything has joints

As I noted in my previous book, *The New Laws of Psychology*, the ancient Greek philosopher Plato once suggested that natural science was the art of 'carving nature at its joints'. Plato said a lot of things, some of which were actually nonsense. What he meant by this particular phrase was that scientists need to identify and classify the phenomena – the birds, animals, plants and insects, the minerals, elements and forces – that shape the natural world. The idea of creating order out of chaos is seductive, and scientists in many branches of science – geology, botany and biology in particular – have always had a strong emphasis on classification.

The process of assigning a mental health 'diagnosis' is essentially one of classification. This kind of classification has a double attraction for psychiatry. Firstly, as a standard methodology within science and medicine, it is pleasingly 'scientific'. Psychiatry, in particular, occasionally appears rather sensitive to accusations of being unscientific. Secondly, for a while, classification appeared to offer some benefit.

Johann Reil first used the term 'psychiatry' in 1808. The 19th century saw huge leaps forward in medical understanding and skills, just as it saw progress across society. One of the particular leaps forward related to the classification of diseases, drawing on new knowledge of physiology and infection and based on scientific principles. The progress in medical practice is undeniable. And early psychiatrists were faced with the same challenges as modern psychiatrists. They were caring for large numbers of very distressed patients with complicated, ever changing, problems in a context of great social change and significant deprivation. The classification and definition of what is now called 'schizophrenia' was largely influenced by the work of the psychiatrist Emil Kraepelin. In 1919, Kraepelin suggested that the confusing and distressing chaos of the problems he was trying to address in his hospital role could be simplified by classifying them into two broad illnesses: 'dementia praecox' (Latin for loss of intelligence before the onset of old-age, a term later replaced by 'schizophrenia') and 'manic-depression'.[2]

We are still living with this legacy. In the field of medical science as applied to physical health, this is a treasure – we are hugely fortunate, today, that doctors can identify infections and pathologies of physiology from their opaque symptoms, aided by diagnostic laboratory tests. But, in my opinion, Plato's dictum does not apply well to problems of human emotion. I accept that 'carving nature at the joints' has great applicability in physical medicine, but Platonic quotes are not always scientifically valid. Plato, for instance, also said that there were three kinds of men (he didn't mention women), men of gold, men of silver and men of bronze. He used this to justify social hierarchies, segregation, exploitation and slavery ... while admitting it was a 'noble lie'. So I don't accept everything Plato says (in fact, I tend to follow the advice of Roger Bacon from the 15th century, who advised people not to follow the advice of those in positions of authority merely because of their station ... and got himself excommunicated as a result). And when we look at the classification of human distress, we need to be equally critical. If classification depends on 'carving nature at its joints', where are those 'joints'? In fact, are there any 'joints' at all? Is it actually ever possible to make those kinds of categorical decisions in the field of mental health? I sometimes use the rather silly analogy of a chicken and a sausage – we can carve a chicken at the joints, but a sausage has no joints. I think mental health is a sausage, not a chicken. It simply doesn't have these joints.

Of course, if psychiatric diagnoses were valid, then the classification of mental disorders could lead to progress, just as it has in physical health. It would allow the causes and origins of real 'disorders' to be understood. If we could reliably and validly identify a group of people with a particular disorder, we could examine their medical status or life histories to reveal a particular brain abnormality, a particular biochemical imbalance, a particular set of experiences or a particular pattern of thinking which could then explain the origins of that particular disorder. Since this has been successful in other branches of medicine, it makes sense to assume it could work in psychiatry. The problem is it just simply doesn't appear to work that way.

## What is 'abnormal' anyway?

In the most 'scientific' of the sciences, physics, we talk about 'universal laws'. These are statements that describe the functioning of the natural world in its most fundamental sense. I commute to work by car and unfortunately drive for quite long distances on motorways. So my journey to work (like, I suppose, everything else in life) depends on the operation of the laws of physics. When it rains, we often see collisions and other accidental tragedies; the roads are slippery, it is harder to see. When people have accidents, the police investigate the probable or likely cause of the incident for legal and insurance purposes. Their analysis includes human factors, but also includes complex physics. To work out why a tragedy has occurred, the investigators will calculate things like the velocity of the vehicles involved, coefficients of friction between rubber and tarmac, reaction times calculated using equations of acceleration and deceleration, the role of centrifugal forces, tyre pressures and 'footprint', the role of aquaplaning, lift, etc. They will measure elements of the physical world; the weight of the vehicles, radius of turns, the slope of ascents or descents, whether the conditions were wet or dry, the temperature, tyre pressures, the condition of brakes and the nature of the road surface. All these aspects of physics are important; they explain why accidents happen. But road traffic investigators don't use a special branch of physics called 'abnormal physics'. We don't expect scientists to apply one special branch of physics to car crashes and differentiate this from the laws of physics that apply to 'normal life'. There is not an 'abnormal coefficient of friction' that leads to car crashes and a 'normal coefficient of friction' that keeps us safe. Instead, and wisely, we recognise that it is important to understand the universal laws of physics – such as friction – and then use that understanding to help design safer roads and to drive more safely as individuals.

The laws of psychology are similarly universal. Psychological principles apply to health and well-being and to distress and problems. There simply isn't an 'abnormal psychology' that applies to distress or explains 'illnesses' and a different 'normal psychology' that applies to everything else. There is just psychology. Everybody makes sense of their world, and does so on the basis of the experiences that they have and the learning that occurs over their lifetime. We all use the same basic processes to understand the world, even if we come to very different conclusions. The patterns and contingencies of reinforcement – rewards and punishments – shape us all: the basic psychology of behavioural learning is universal. We all learn to repeat those things that are reinforcing, and we all withdraw from things that cause us pain. We all construct more or less useful frameworks for understanding the world, and we all use those frameworks to predict the future and guide our actions. That's true for someone who has learned to trust people, and it's true for someone who has learned to distrust them. Middle-aged people from the UK will remember Eric Morecombe on the piano saying that he's playing 'all the right notes... just not necessarily in the right order'. As I'm writing this book, I'm using common words and the standard 26 letters of the alphabet, but hopefully I'm putting them together in a novel sequence. So it is with our learning about the world and how that learning affects our emotions. We're all using the same processes of learning and understanding, and those processes have similar effects on our behaviour and emotions. However, because no one is exactly the same as anyone else, or has exactly the same experiences, we all make sense of the world in slightly different ways, with different consequences. But that's entirely different from suggesting that there is some kind of 'abnormal psychology'.

So I believe that we all share one psychology; it's wrong to separate 'normal' from 'abnormal'. But it's also true that we can't make that separation in our everyday experience. There's a frequently quoted statistic that mental health problems will affect one in four of us in our lifetimes. It's often used to campaign for greater understanding and greater funding. But it's a curious statistic. We ALL have mental health problems. We ALL get anxious or depressed from time to time, hear our names mentioned when nobody's said anything. So we all – ALL – have mental health, and we all have mental health problems. The real question is, how severe, how long-standing, how distressing are those problems? The 'one-in-four' statistic may be misleading and distracting, as it gives the impression that there are two groups of people: those with mental health problems and those without. It refers to the number of people whose problems would meet the diagnostic criteria for a mental health problem.[3] Given that mental health professionals seem to be lunging headlong towards labelling everything and everybody, that statistic is meaningless. Except... it illustrates how common these problems are. And that's important.

Even complex, difficult, distressing and perplexing psychotic experiences are very common in the general population. Many, many people hold beliefs that others consider strange or bizarre (for example, belief in UFOs, alien abduction, ghosts or telepathy). We all feel suspicious of other people from time to time. It's a standing joke that professors all think that their academic colleagues are out to get them (of course it's because we know that they are!). The extreme state that we call 'paranoia' or 'persecutory delusions' is on a continuum with these feelings of suspiciousness. There is natural variance between people in this respect. We've all had different experiences and we have different reasons why we might have become distrusting or suspicious. We all know people who are 'touchy' in this respect. And we've all been in situations where it makes sense to be particularly vigilant (walking down an inner city street at night, for example) and in such situations it is easy to be frightened by even the most innocent things.

So it's not surprising that surveys of the general population routinely reveal that somewhere between 10% and 15% of people have had a hallucination at some point in their lives. Although only about one person in a hundred receives a formal diagnosis of 'schizophrenia', surveys suggest that 'psychotic-like' experiences are as much as 50 times more common than this. This means that perhaps half of us have heard or seen things that aren't there, have been convinced by things that other people regard as strange or bizarre, or have been unreasonably suspicious of other people. We know that extreme circumstances, such as sensory or sleep deprivation, can lead to paranoia and hallucinations. And there are many people who have strange experiences (such as visions, auditory hallucinations, or profound spiritual experiences) but interpret them as spiritually enriching. Different cultures have very different expectations in terms of what is considered normal, as well as hugely different ways of describing things. In many cultures, it is routine to describe dead people being present with you in day-to-day life. Some of the differences are to do with use of language: people describe similar experiences differently and the same words (or their nearest translations) can mean something else in another culture. But different cultures also have fundamentally different beliefs as to what constitute the 'symptoms of mental illness' as opposed to normal experiences or religious and spiritual experiences (such as the presence of ancestors, the everyday tangible presence of God, the effects of divine intercession or spirit possession). In some cultures, things that the West sees as problems are seen as spiritual gifts to be respected and protected, for example Shamen or mediums. Although psychotic experiences can sometimes be extremely distressing and disabling, for other people, they may even be life enhancing. For some people, they are both at different times, or even perhaps at the same time.

At this point in the argument, my colleagues (both psychologists and psychiatrists) often point out that a diagnostic approach is useful because there are very significant differences between 'real' problems that are 'hugely distressing' and the normal ups and downs of everyday life. That is absolutely true. We all get miserable from time to time. When things go wrong in my life – when a relationship fails, or I fail at work or someone close to me is seriously ill – I (and we all) sometimes feel low, unmotivated, have problems sleeping etc. (i.e., experience some of the so-called symptoms of depression). I am not, of course, claiming that is in any sense as serious a problem – is the same problem – as somebody who has been depressed for years, has harmed themselves, is reliant on medication and is contemplating taking their own life. But I am saying that the experiences and emotions lie on a continuum. Many important things, life-threatening things, lie on continua. Many of us, these days, are overweight. Some people could do with losing a few pounds, but some people are in serious and acute danger. These issues lie on continua, but it does not follow that, because there is a continuum of experiences, that the one extreme is somehow no longer being differentiated from the other. My boss, the Vice-Chancellor, earns a very great deal more than the cleaners at my university (he earns quite a lot more than me). Clearly, salary is something that lies on a continuum (you just keep adding £10 notes one after the other for a very long time), but nobody is saying that this is equivalent to saying that everybody earns the same amount. So the distressing and life-threatening experiences that fall under the umbrella of 'mental health problems' are serious, real and occasionally life threatening. But they aren't unique and different parts of the human experience. They lie on continua with other common experiences, and the same psychological principles apply.

## Why, and how, do we diagnose 'mental illnesses'?

Many people mistakenly believe that psychiatric diagnoses reflect real 'illnesses'; things that 'really' exist. Scientific analysis of the problems that people experience and their relationship to these diagnostic labels suggests that this is an error. Some people do find diagnostic labels reassuring or helpful because they appear to recognise, explain and validate their problems, and (currently at least) often qualify people for help. Some professionals and policy-makers mistakenly assume that we need to use diagnoses in order to allocate resources to those who need them. However, other services – for example many public and social services – achieve this without the need for 'diagnoses'. Many medical and legal professionals, and in particular medical researchers, mistakenly believe that diagnoses are needed in order to allow people to communicate efficiently with one another. However I would argue that here again they are misleading and unnecessary; a simple and direct list of a person's actual experiences and problems would provide more information and communicate much more than a diagnostic label. Of course we need to research into the nature, causes and remedies of problems, but again that does not mean that diagnosis is necessary; I'll explain shortly why researchers would be better advised to study the nature of, causes of and proper response to specific, easily identified problems rather than looking for differences between groups of people with different 'diagnoses'. In order to understand the extent to which psychiatric diagnoses are mistaken and unhelpful we need to look at how 'mental illness' is currently classified. There are two major international classificatory systems for the classification and diagnosis of mental health problems:

## The World Health Organization's International Standard Classification of Diseases, Injuries and Causes of Death – ICD-10

One of the first actions of the World Health Organization, immediately after its formation in 1948, was to publish a comprehensive list of the world's diseases and illnesses. The International Standard Classification of Diseases, Injuries and Causes of Death (or 'ICD'), predictably included psychological and psychiatric 'conditions'. This effectively ensured that these kinds of problems were seen as the responsibility of medicine and ensured that diagnosis, classification and categorisation was the method of choice. This diagnostic manual has been extensively revised over the years, and we are now using ICD-10, the tenth and most recent revision.[4] ICD-10 is, technically at least, the international standard classification system, recommended for administrative and epidemiological purposes and forms the basis of statistical procedures in the UK National Health Service.

## American Psychiatric Association's Diagnostic and Statistical Manual – DSM-5

The immediate post-war period also saw the publication of the American Psychiatric Association's Diagnostic and Statistical Manual – DSM.[5] This was based on the administrative scheme used by the US Army in World War II. As with ICD, the DSM system has been revised and re-edited over time, meaning that the current edition is the fifth – DSM-5. The DSM franchise is, of course, very widely used in the USA. Because DSM is used for research classification as well as epidemiological and statistical purposes, and because most researchers want to publish their results in US-based, English language publications, it has become standard practice for researchers, even in Europe, to use DSM criteria. The two systems, ICD and DSM, have run in parallel ever since and there is considerable overlap, and increasing convergence, between the two systems.

The fact that there are two separate classification systems is somewhat embarrassing for the diagnostic model. It is embarrassing because if there is an objective illness of 'depression' (or 'schizophrenia' or 'attention deficit hyperactivity disorder' or whatever) it would seem odd if social factors such as whether we follow an American or European tradition were to determine its existence. Scientists and clinicians recognise this, and one of the principal reasons for the latest revision of DSM (from DSM-IV to become DSM-5) was to permit easier 'read-across' between the two systems. There are even mechanisms for translating DSM codes into ICD codes. However, the two codes are not identical. A good illustration of this is in the diagnostic criteria for depression – which is, of course, very common indeed. The DSM-5 diagnostic guidelines are more complex, more detailed and more prescriptive than the ICD-10 criteria. It is possible for a person to meet the ICD-10 criteria for a diagnosis of depression, but fail to meet the DSM-5 criteria. For example, if you have been experiencing low mood, a loss of interest and enjoyment and reduced energy for the past three weeks, you would meet the ICD-10 criteria for a diagnosis of 'depressive episode'. But unless you are also experiencing weight loss or sleep disturbance, feel agitated, worthless or guilty, are unable to concentrate or having thoughts of suicide, you would not qualify for the equivalent DSM-5 diagnosis of 'major depressive episode'. That might be rare (many people who meet the ICD-10 criteria will, in fact, meet the DSM-5 criteria), but illustrates some of the confusion.

There have been many specific changes as DSM-IV has been revised to become DSM-5. One controversial change[6] was the decision to drop a specific exclusion criterion. The fourth edition suggested that people should not be diagnosed with 'major depression' if they had been recently bereaved. In technical language, it was not appropriate to record a diagnosis of 'major depressive episode' if (in technical language) '…the symptoms are not better accounted for by Bereavement…'. We all feel low when a loved one has died and so, the logic went, we don't need to label people in that situation as 'ill'. But this requirement was dropped in DSM-5. That means it now *is* possible to receive a diagnosis of 'major depressive episode' if you experience low mood following the death of a loved one. Many people worldwide were concerned by this development and the idea that someone grieving for a loved one could be diagnosed with a 'mental illness'. I agree. But here are – within, strictly within, the logic of psychiatric diagnosis – reasons for this odd decision. First, the ICD-10 doesn't have an exclusion for bereavement, so it could be argued that this brings the two manuals closer together. And, technically – and this will be a surprise to some people – diagnostic manuals are not concerned with the causes of or reasons for a person's problems. If a person is experiencing low mood, they are experiencing low mood. The fact that a loved one has died is a very good reason for such low mood, but it doesn't mean the low mood isn't there.

In my opinion, then, the problem is not really whether bereavement is, or is not, included as an exclusion criterion for a diagnosis of 'major depressive episode'. My concern is a larger one. I simply don't think we should be asking these kinds of questions in the first place.

## Reliability

For a scientist, the first test of a diagnostic system is to ask if it is reliable. To be reliable (in this context), a diagnostic system would need to ensure that two people would both agree on which diagnosis to use. Although people do change over time, a reliable diagnostic system would also mean that the same decision – the same diagnosis – would be assigned again if you repeated the assessment. If a diagnostic system were reliable, we would get the same result each time. One of the reasons that the diagnostic manuals (DSM and ICD) were developed in the first place, and one of the reasons they have been revised, is to ensure reliability. Several years ago, research suggested that clinicians in different countries (the researchers particularly studied the USA and UK) tended to make rather different diagnoses when presented with identical sets of problems.[7] What would lead to a diagnosis of, say 'schizophrenia' in one country would lead to a diagnosis of say 'bipolar disorder' if you were to consult with a clinician in another country. While there are clearly lots of reasons why this might happen (the people reporting the problems might behave differently or say different things, the person making the diagnosis might interview people in a different manner, the environment might be different, etc.), but a central issue was that different countries tended to have different diagnostic systems – different rules for combining symptoms and different systems of naming the 'disorders' that were diagnosed. The DSM and ICD diagnostic systems were drafted specifically to address these kinds of problems; the issue of reliability was addressed by international agreement on criteria, and rules for which 'symptoms' would count towards which diagnosis.

Another way that people tried to improve reliability was by using standardised interviews. In such interviews, a person is asked standard questions about their experiences, with very little deviation from the prepared script. Although the interviews can sometimes be a little stilted, reliability is improved and this is the reason that such interviews are often used in research projects. However, it is rather different in routine clinical practice. In practice, clinicians seldom use such standardised interviews. In any event, the subject matter of psychiatric diagnoses is usually subjective reports of behaviours, thoughts and emotions. These can almost never be independently verified (which is why, incidentally, the legal reports of psychiatrists and psychologists tend to use the phrase '...she reported that...' very frequently. We can't claim to know what she thought, all we can say is what she *said* she thought). So, when we make these sorts of decisions, we have to ask questions about personal experiences and it is often a matter of some judgment as to whether (in the words of DSM-5) they 'cause clinically significant distress or impairment in social, occupational, or other important areas of functioning.'

There are three important things to note here. Firstly, although these diagnostic manuals have improved the reliability of psychiatric diagnosis considerably, it is still rather poor. In fact, reliability appears to be getting progressively worse with each new edition of DSM.[8] Secondly, as fans of psychiatric diagnosis sometimes point out, the reliability of some diagnoses in the arena of physical health is also poor. So, for example, pathologists may be mistaken about the cause of death on as much as a third of occasions when their expert judgements are compared with the results of post-mortems, and even diagnoses of illnesses like tonsillitis can be less reliable than those for 'schizophrenia'. However, there is one important difference: in the arena of physical health, post-mortem examinations and laboratory tests can confirm or refute clinical impressions. There are no such laboratory tests for mental health problems.[9]

And this raises a third issue. Even if psychiatric diagnoses were reliable, that wouldn't be enough. Diagnoses also need to be 'valid' – that is, to be meaningful and to represent real 'things'.

## Validity

It is quite possible for a diagnosis to be completely reliable, but still not be valid. For example, we might suggest that there exists a disorder called 'Kinderman Syndrome'. Kinderman Syndrome might be diagnosed if someone possesses all of the following 'symptoms': having thinning brown hair, a south-east English accent and protruding ears. This diagnosis would probably be quite reliable. Although some interviewers might be poor at discerning a 'south-east English' accent, and some might be uncertain as to the exact definition of 'thinning' hair, I suspect a rigorous investigation would establish that any panel of suitably selected and trained clinicians would be able to agree at least 75% of the time as to whether these criteria are met. We might have to develop the criteria carefully – we might have to define 'protruding' in relation to ears, and even define the exact shade of 'brown' we meant. So there might be some work needed to refine the definitions, and we might need to train our clinicians. But I suspect we could get high reliability.

But is it valid? Is there in any real sense a syndrome, a disorder, a mental illness that – validly – exists merely because we can define it? Of course not. I am sure many of the people I have encountered in my professional life would leap at the idea of 'Kinderman Syndrome'. But we cannot accept that 'mental illnesses' exist merely because we can name them. We can't accept that reliability alone makes a 'disorder' a valid concept.

This is not just a theoretical argument. I mentioned the tragic and scandalous case of Alan Turing earlier in this chapter. Leaving aside the fact that it is immensely difficult reliably to define either heterosexual or homosexual sex (many men who have sex with other men do not regard themselves as gay, and many men who regard themselves as heterosexual have had sexual experiences with other men) the point is that to define somebody as having a 'disorder' because they have sexual preferences that a particular community chooses to repudiate does not make it a valid diagnosis. Incidentally (because I mentioned sexual preference), modern diagnostic manuals do not tend to label sexual preferences as 'disorders'. But they certainly do label distress associated with sexual issues as 'disorders'. So we have 'gender identity disorder'; rather than simply saying that someone has experienced a great deal of distress living in a discriminatory and heterosexist world, we label this distress as a 'disorder'.

There have been plenty of invalid diagnoses – diagnoses that psychiatrists have unhesitatingly rejected. In the 19th century, an American doctor called Samuel Cartwright seriously suggested that slaves who attempted to escape from their captors were suffering from the illness of 'drapetomania'[10] (the Greek word drapetes means a runaway slave). According to Cartwright, men and women with a desire for freedom were merely exhibiting the symptom of an illness. In a frightening reflection of the behaviour of academics and clinicians, Cartwright wrote a scientific paper (the 'diseases and peculiarities of the negro race') in which he hypothesised that the aetiology of his newly identified 'illness' involved slave-owners treating their possessions as if they were human beings. Unsurprisingly, Cartwright suggested that the 'treatment' for 'drapetomania' was whipping.

Of course, not only is this nonsense, it was recognised as such by the psychiatrists of the day. But ... those psychiatrists did not suggest that it was equally nonsensical to medicalise a person's sexual preference. In my professional opinion, we need to question the validity of all mental health diagnoses. As colleagues and I said in a recent paper – we should 'drop the language of disorder'.[11]

## 'Oppositional defiant disorder' ... really?

Many people unfamiliar with psychiatric diagnostic practices are surprised to learn that the DSM-5 includes a diagnosis of 'oppositional defiant disorder'. This diagnosis, used with children, is defined by 'a pattern of negativistic, hostile, and defiant behaviour lasting at least 6 months'. The specific diagnostic criteria include: actively defying or refusing to comply with adults' requests or rules, deliberately annoying people, blaming other people for his or her mistakes or misbehaviour and being angry and resentful. If you believe DSM-5 (I don't), these can be grouped into three types: angry/irritable mood, argumentative/defiant behaviour, and vindictiveness.

Children can sometimes be painfully unhappy. And children can sometimes be entirely unresponsive to their parents, or, indeed to other authority figures. I certainly would not want to imply that such problems don't exist or that they are trivial. I just don't think they are 'illnesses'. I am – to be clear – absolutely convinced that children and young people can be negativistic. They can be hostile. They can actively refuse to comply with adults' requests or rules. I have to say, these kinds of problems are often indications that the child has experienced some significant trauma. But in any case, I do not wish to make light of real, painful, problems. These kinds of difficulties can have terrible consequences for children and their parents. But I simply don't think it's sensible, useful, scientifically appropriate or clinically justifiable to suggest that the children have a 'disorder'. Apart from anything else, this kind of labelling makes people think that these problems are not really normal human problems at all, but instead are 'symptoms of mental illness'. I don't like it when my children are defiant or refuse to comply with my requests. But I don't think they are mentally ill.

Another example of the problems with the idea of 'mental illnesses' is the contentious issue of 'personality disorder'. 'Personality disorders' are defined as 'long-standing patterns of maladaptive behaviour that constitute immature and inappropriate ways of coping with stress or solving problems'. It is fascinating and horrible how a person's whole character can be rendered into a 'disorder'. Examples of personality disorder include; 'antisocial personality disorder', 'paranoid personality disorder', 'narcissistic personality disorder', 'schizoid personality disorder' etc. Antisocial personality disorder is particularly interesting in the context of the validity of diagnoses of mental disorder, because it illustrates the weird circularity of these ideas. Do people do bad things because they are suffering from 'antisocial personality disorder' or do they get labelled with 'antisocial personality disorder' because they do bad things?

'Personality disorders' are interesting in part because the authors of diagnostic manuals seem to be entirely undecided as to how many of these 'disorders' there are – DSM-5 and ICD-10 do not agree. Discussions and debates frequently occur as to whether 'personality disorders' could be entirely expunged from the diagnostic manuals (replaced, perhaps, with a description of personality traits). So they appear to have a fleeting, ghost-like reality – written into existence; potentially deleted – as the committees deliberate. But, despite their oddity, their circularity, their tenuous claimed validity, it can be significant if you receive a diagnosis of 'personality disorder'. The UK Government linked an entire offender management programme – the Dangerous and Severe Personality Disorder programme, designed to help manage very seriously dangerous offenders – to the concept.

## On being sane in insane places

The 1973 experiment by David Rosenhan – 'on being sane in insane places'[12] – has been widely reported. But it bears repetition. Rosenhan arranged for eight ordinary people from conventional backgrounds to go to hospitals in the USA and tell unsuspecting psychiatrists that they had heard disembodied voices saying 'empty', 'hollow' or 'thud'. Apart from reporting this experience (which is, of course, a conventional criterion for the diagnosis of schizophrenia), the eight undercover researchers were told to reply to all questions honestly.

All eight of them were admitted to hospital, the majority of them with a diagnosis of schizophrenia. Once they were admitted, each 'pseudopatient' behaved normally. But the fact that they had been admitted to hospital and given a psychiatric diagnosis appeared to change the way they were regarded by the staff. Staff saw one pseudopatient pacing the corridors – they were bored – and suggested that they were experiencing 'anxiety' when seen. One pseudopatient was seen to be writing – in fact, writing notes of their experiences – which was recorded as 'patient engages in writing behaviour'. The scientific or medicalised language ('writing behaviour') subtly indicates that something odd is going on. Rosenhan reports that it was only the other patients in the hospital who realised that there was something odd going on; one challenged a researcher, saying: 'you're not crazy, you're a journalist or a professor. You're checking up on the hospital.'

Sadly, the treatment that the pseudopatients received in hospital was deeply worrying. Once in hospital, the undercover researchers reported that they no longer heard any voices. And indeed, after an average of 19 days (with a range of 7 to 52), the staff agreed that they were now well enough to be discharged – all were discharged with a diagnosis of schizophrenia in remission. But, by then, the pseudopatients had been prescribed a total of 2100 pills. We should be careful not to read too much into Rosenhan's research. It was conducted in 1973 and things have undoubtedly changed. But we should note that staff members only spent 11% of their time interacting with patients in Rosenhan's study, and that comments like 'Come on, you mother f – – -s, get out of bed' were reported as common. We should contrast this with the stories we are told about residential mental health units today, some of which I have included in this book.

Many people argue that it's possible to read a little too much into Rosenhan's study. For me, however, this study is important. For example, I think that, within the logic of the 'disease model' of psychiatric diagnosis, the psychiatrists apparently duped by Rosenhan's pseudopatients had reasonable grounds for making their diagnostic decisions – and subsequent decisions to admit to hospital and prescribe medication. In the standard diagnostic manuals, hearing voices – experiencing auditory hallucinations – is a symptom of 'schizophrenia'. And the disease model dictates to psychiatrists that 'schizophrenia' warrants hospital treatment and medication. Within this (flawed) system, diagnosis, classification, hospitalisation and prescription are justified. My point is that I don't believe the 'disease model' is appropriate, and so the diagnostic and treatment decisions that follow are equally flawed.

## A tool for action

Many psychologists as well as psychiatrists see some merits in the diagnostic approach. About a third of the people involved in the taskforce drawing up DSM-5 were psychologists. For many, their decision to accept a diagnostic approach is purely practical – they see DSM as a tool for categorising problems and suggesting what might help. In the next chapter, we will examine some of the evidence concerning the extent to which diagnoses are useful in assisting treatment decisions. In short, I believe diagnoses are unhelpful.

As we shall see in the next chapter, it is very difficult to predict what treatments people will find helpful on the basis of the diagnosis they receive. In physical medicine, specific types of drugs are helpful for specific problems. For example, penicillin is a specific treatment for bacterial infection and not for viral infection. It is different with psychiatric medication. Although you might imagine that the drugs known as 'antipsychotics' are specific treatments for 'schizophrenia', this is not the case. Not all people with a diagnosis of 'schizophrenia' benefit significantly. At the same time, some people with other diagnoses do seem to benefit from these drugs. If you are experiencing a manic episode, for example, you may find that 'antipsychotic' medication offers some temporary respite. This is not what you would expect if 'bipolar disorder' were 'carved at the joints' from 'schizophrenia'. Proponents of diagnoses usually stress that diagnosis is needed to decide the right treatment. But in reality psychiatric diagnosis appears almost irrelevant in this regard and some psychiatrists, notably Dr Joanna Moncrieff, suggest that diagnosis should not be used as a basis for prescribing. This seems a rather fatal problem for the diagnostic approach.

Diagnoses also appear to have little practical utility when it comes to prognosis. A valid diagnosis, a diagnosis that means something in the real world, should say something about the outcome that people given the diagnosis should expect. Again, however (with the exception of neurological diseases and learning disability, which are rather different) the outcomes for people given nearly every diagnosis are highly variable. Moreover, each person's outcome appears dependent much more on their social situation than on their diagnosis – so whether they are in a relationship, whether they have friends, whether they have a job, whether they have somewhere decent to live. Health care professionals, quite correctly, tell people that there are a huge range of possible outcomes, and (again correctly) that many things can be done to affect their prognosis. Arguably this all makes diagnosis rather redundant.

There is a perception that people with psychiatric diagnoses are more likely than others to be violent. However, in fact, very few acts of violence are committed by people with a history of mental health problems. The most important factors predicting violence are: having a history of violence, being male and using alcohol. Specific diagnoses like 'schizophrenia' do not predict dangerousness. Some specific experiences and beliefs, such as a conviction that others intend to do you physical harm, or hearing voices telling you to do something violent, are associated with a small increased risk. But even among people who have these experiences, few actually end up acting on them. Even where people do, the association is with the specific experiences or beliefs rather than with a particular diagnosis. Despite this story of failure, many of my colleagues who advocate the use of diagnosis in mental health care appear still to rely on the myth of utility – the idea that diagnoses are useful. One (medically-qualified) contributor to an on-line blog (hosted by the well-respected Oxford University Press) tried to defuse this row by saying that: 'clinicians need to communicate to each other, and even a wrong diagnosis allows them to do so.' This is not only foolish, it's dangerous. It suggests not only that clinicians can permit their care to be guided by 'wrong' diagnoses, but they should (perhaps need to) share their errors with colleagues. Another contributor suggested that we need to regard diagnoses such as schizophrenia as 'heterogeneous diagnoses'. So we have one influential proponent suggesting that diagnoses are useful even if they are 'wrong', and another suggesting that they can be catch-all or 'heterogeneous'. Whilst it seems very strange to suggest that something that is wrong can also be necessary, it is truer to say that psychiatric diagnoses are 'heterogeneous'; research suggests that they simply do not represent discrete phenomena.

## Statistical relationships are not diagnoses

Scientists have applied powerful statistical techniques to try to understand whether people's experiences of mental health problems do cluster together in the way predicted by the diagnostic approach. The central idea of diagnosis is that particular psychological problems cluster together. Diagnosis depends on a particular 'disorder' or 'illness' having shared characteristics that make it distinct from other 'disorders' or 'illnesses'. But in general the results of this approach have not been supportive of the diagnostic model. There do appear to be patterns and relationships between problems (of which more later) but these relationships tend to cut across diagnostic categories.

It is important to note that this applies – perhaps more powerfully – when we explore the role of biological factors. It was with some fanfare that researchers announced[13] that they had identified some genetic factors associated with a range of common mental health problems. It is important, and significant, work. But these genetic characteristics, the associated biochemical pathways and the psychological processes that affect and are affected by them, are not specific to particular diagnoses. Quite the reverse, the biological and psychological pathways quite clearly cut across these diagnostic categories.

## There is no 'normal' and 'abnormal' in mental health

The idea that there is a quintessential distinction between normal emotions and 'mental illness' is widespread. People talk about 'clinical depression' to distinguish it from 'ordinary' depression. One influential journalist in the field of popular science recently decried how people fail to distinguish everyday feelings of depression from (real) 'depressive symptoms'. The disease model of mental health tends to reinforce the idea that the experiences and emotions of people whose problems are placed in diagnostic categories such as 'depression', 'schizophrenia' and 'bipolar disorder' are qualitatively different from 'normal' emotions and experiences. And this faces us with a real contrast. Traditional psychiatry, the 'disease model' of mental health and the diagnostic approach all conceptualise, or at least present a vision of, 'mental illnesses' as qualitatively different to and separable from normality. Research suggests something rather different: that there is no dividing line between 'normal' and 'abnormal' emotions, experiences or behaviours.

Many people, especially clinical psychologists, have suggested that these supposed 'symptoms' of mental illnesses in fact lie on a continuum with normality. Sometimes experiences and emotions become problematical, but this is the same with anything else: any human experience or tendency can become a problem if it is extreme. This idea is neither new nor unusual. I opened this chapter with a short quote from Herman Mellville's novel *Billy Budd*. It is worthwhile reproducing it at slightly greater length:

> Who in the rainbow can draw the line where the violet tint ends and the orange tint begins? Distinctly we see the difference of the colors, but where exactly does the one first blendingly enter into the other? So with sanity and insanity. In pronounced cases there is no question about them. But in some supposed cases, in various degrees supposedly

less pronounced, to draw the exact line of demarkation few will under-take tho' for a fee some professional experts will. There is nothing nameable but that some men will undertake to do it for pay.[14]

An editorial in the Times from 1854 expresses it equally eloquently:

> Nothing can be more slightly defined than the line of demarcation between sanity and insanity. Physicians and lawyers have vexed them-selves with attempts at definitions in a case where definition is impos-sible. There has never yet been given to the world anything in the shape of a formula upon this subject which may not be torn to shreds in five minutes by any ordinary logician. Make the definition too narrow, it becomes meaningless; make it too wide, the whole human race are involved in the drag-net. In strictness, we are all mad as often as we give way to passion, to prejudice, to vice to vanity; but if all the passionate, prejudiced, vicious, and vain people in this world are to be locked up as lunatics, who is to keep the keys to the asylum?[15]

I agree. I cannot see how we can draw 'a line of demarcation between sanity and insanity'. I can see why the idea that there is such a dividing line is popular: it reassures us that mental health problems are discrete, diagnosable entities, experienced by people who are different to us. But in truth, all these experiences lie on continua.

This continuum approach is best understood by thinking about common experiences such as anxiety. All of us will have experienced anxiety at some point in our lives. Some of us have experienced sheer terror, or perhaps become extremely anxious very frequently. Many more of us are often anxious, but to a lesser degree. Only a minority of us will ever experience extremes of anxiety such as a series of panic attacks, crippling obsessions or compulsions to do certain things that would be recognised in the diagnostic textbooks as justifying a diagnosis of an anxiety 'disorder'. Many of us will have had unusual perceptual experi-ences from time to time, but most of us will have not been disturbed by them and dismissed them as transient and trivial events. Others are plagued by continual psychosis. Some people hear disembodied voices, but regard the experience as 'normal'. Other people are terrified by what they hear. We all feel low from time to time, but some people feel so bad that they contemplate suicide. And – and this is important – all shades of experience fall in between.

Madness and sanity are not qualitatively different states of mind, but should instead be seen as lying at the extreme ends of several spectra of experience. In fact, sanity cannot really be seen as occupying the oppo-site end to madness on any realistic 'normal' spectrum of experience. If we imagine madness at one end of a continuum, the opposite end will be a never-experienced utopia where we are gloriously happy, rational at all times, clear-sighted and with the acute and precise hearing of an owl, and, in the words of the Times editor, free from all passion, prejudice, vice and vanity.

The editor of the *Times* also pointed out another fundamental truth that I am attempting to express. The factors that lead to madness are aspects of normal psychology. The *Times* editorial states that we are all mad so long as we give way to passion, prejudice, vice and vanity. These are – in the slightly poetic prose of a Victorian journalist – normal psychological processes. If passion, prejudice etc., change how we think about the world, then we will blur the lines that separate 'sanity' from 'insanity'.

These continua are not necessarily simple, straight-line, relation-ships. Part of the way that psychologists understand a wide range of mental health problems is based on understanding vicious cycles and feedback loops. When something bad happens – maybe somebody passes on a piece of bad news – we tend to feel a little low. The way that human memories work means that, when our mood drops, it makes it more likely that we think about more negative things. That is simple psychology, that's how a lot of advertising works. If we can sow a seed of an idea in somebody's mind, the network of associations will lead them to think of a wide range of related matters. So, after bad news, it's very easy to begin to experience a snowball of negative memories. This might lead us to feel even worse, and perhaps to interpret subsequent events in a more negative light than we would do otherwise. Those interpretations in turn might drive our mood down further. When we become depressed, we feel fatigued, lethargic and 'anhedonic' (we are no longer enjoying things we used to). It is then natural to withdraw – to withdraw from social events, to stop doing those things we used to do (but which we no longer enjoy so much), to let our self-care slip. When we do that, we are cutting ourselves off from things that offer us the possibility of reward and enjoyment. And so, our mood drops further. And a vicious cycle ensues, pulling us down into depression. Many problems that involve anxiety also show these kinds of feedback loops. If we are anxious about something (performing in public, perhaps) it is very tempting, very reassuring, very easy, to avoid situations that might expose us to our fears (we might decide to take the day off when our line-manager invites a theatre group to offer a 'mythodrama' session – and, yes, I was once exposed to 'mythodrama' as part of a training course!). That makes us feel better, feel less anxious…temporarily. But it can lead to further, deeper problems. If, for example, we deal with the impending mythodrama visit (or, more precisely, with our intrusive and obsessive anxious thoughts about that visit) by deploying some compulsive rituals that make us less anxious (wearing our lucky socks, for example) we can find that we become effectively addicted to the compulsions to cope with future anxiety. The fact that many emotional problems are driven at least in part by such vicious cycles means that our journey along the pathway – down the continuum – is not a linear progression. Once we start, we can accelerate progressively downwards…like a snowball, as we roll downhill, we pick up speed and our problems can escalate. So you can see how normal psychological processes can lead to a wide variety of sometimes quite extreme experiences and states.

We can see continua in every area of mental health and well-being. Children differ in their ability to learn, to pay attention at school, to focus their attention and to regulate their emotions. For parents, these are all part of the business of childhood, of parenting, of education. When I was a child, I was unable to remain focussed and attentive for the full range of the school day and into the evening. I wasn't one of the worst in this regard – I managed to concentrate well enough to do OK at school and go to university – but my attentiveness was certainly not 100%. Even now, I am still distracted by squirrels outside the window, by conversations in the corridor, by the nagging suspicion that there is something interesting down by the coffee machine. It is simply an inevitable part of the human condition that some of us have more difficulty than others. Occasionally children's problems with concentration cause their parents and teachers great concern. Sometimes these difficulties cause real disruption to school life. Unsurprisingly, such problems tend to be associated with other problems and difficulties. Equally unsurprisingly, there is a wide range of biological and social factors that can affect a child's ability to concentrate. But all that is hugely different to the way in which we currently often approach these problems – by invoking the idea of an 'illness' called 'attention deficit hyperactivity disorder' or 'ADHD' which only some children 'suffer from'. As Sami Timimi (who is, incidentally a child and adolescent psychiatrist) and Jonathan Leo have eloquently argued, we should not think of these things as 'illnesses', or even worse 'diseases'.[16]

The recent publication of DSM-5 (the fifth edition of the franchise) in 2013, galvanised into action many of us who believe that diagnosing putative diseases is an inappropriate basis for high quality mental health care. The most recent revision of the American diagnostic system saw the lowering of a swathe of diagnostic thresholds. This will have the effect of inflating the apparent prevalence of mental health problems in the general population. Just as when politicians re-define key statistics, millions more people across the world could be regarded as 'having a mental disorder', not because circumstances have made them more distressed, or because there has been a fall in resilience, but merely because the criteria have been changed. This might be good news for pharmaceutical companies, but it is a threat to the rest of us and especially to vulnerable populations such as children and older people. It makes statistics something of a nonsense, as any epidemiological data are dependent on the whim of committees. But more importantly, we all, and particularly people who use mental health services, are harmed by the continued and continuous medicalisation of their natural and understandable responses to their experiences. These responses undoubtedly have distressing consequences, and the people affected need help and support. But even extreme experiences are better understood as normal individual variation than as illnesses.

The changes in the 2013 revision of DSM-5 represent an increased emphasis on the supposed biological underpinnings of psychological distress; the language is couched in terms of biological illness. This is also worrying, since it does not reflect the widespread scientific consensus that distressing experiences are the result of complex, individual interactions between biological, social and psychological factors rather than the result of a disease process. By using the language of 'disorder', diagnostic manuals (and DSM-5 is merely the latest and possibly the worst example) undermine a humane response; they imply that these experiences are the product of an underlying biological defect. The publication of DSM-5 in 2013 provoked something of a minor revolution. We saw the growth of a significant community of opposition drawn from a range of groups. Psychiatrists, psychologists, scientists and users of mental health services alike voiced their opposition to many of its proposals and particularly the pathologising of grief.[17] When someone close to us dies, many of us suffer profound, long-lasting, grief. That is not an illness, it's the price we pay for love. War is traumatic – experiences of conflict change the way we see the world and our part in it, and the traumatically emotional memories are encoded in our minds in ways that cause understandable problems into the future. But it is not a 'disorder' to remain distressed by bereavement after three months or to be traumatised by the experience of industrialised military conflict. Our children need to learn how to manage their emotions, to attend to their studies sufficiently to learn, and to grow up with a sense of moral and social responsibility. It is undeniably a problem – for the children, for their parents, for teachers and for society – when that goes wrong. We need to offer help. But it isn't an 'illness'.

This does not – absolutely not – mean that I, and those colleagues who share my views, believe the problems do not exist. It does not mean that we consider them to be trivial. There are many social problems that are not illnesses. Debt and crime are not illnesses. Of course we need to understand how and why children can manage their emotions and focus their attention. We need to study the neuroscience of these phenomena just as much as we need to study the social and cultural aspects. But they are not 'illnesses'.

## If we don't diagnose, what's the alternative?

We need a wholesale revision of the way we think about psychological distress. We should recognise that distress is an unfortunate but nevertheless normal, not abnormal, part of human life. People experience many difficult circumstances in their lives, and often become distressed as a result. This needs to be reflected in the way we identify, describe and respond to that distress. We also need to acknowledge the overwhelming evidence that severe distress or unusual experiences (which now attract the misleading label of 'psychiatric symptoms') lie at one end of continua with less unusual and distressing mental states. That means there is no easy 'cut-off' between 'normal' experience and 'mental health problems'.

Some people obviously feel that diagnostic labels are helpful. They say that is important for them to learn that their problems have a name. But in reality, this sense that a diagnosis is helpful or reassuring cannot come from any greater understanding of the problems, any better knowledge of their causes or aetiology, appropriate treatment or prognosis – because diagnoses simply can't offer that information. Instead, the sense of helpfulness seems to result from the person knowing that they have been listened to (and heard), that their problems have been recognised (in both senses of the word), understood, validated, that these problems can be explained (and are themselves explicable rather than simply 'mad') and that some help can be offered. In the flawed world of present-day services, however, people often find that they are reassured by (or at least accept) a diagnosis, feel some immediate reassurance, but then find any real help is illusory. The diagnoses convey very limited useful information, will not explain things, will not guide treatment and will not help predict the future. Instead, a clear description of a person's real problems would be much more useful. A description of an individual's actual problems would provide more information and be of greater communicative value than any diagnostic label.

## Simply list the problems ... with some scientific specificity

A perfectly appropriate alternative to diagnosis would be simply to list a person's problems. A simple list of problems (properly defined) would be more than sufficient as a basis for individual care planning, for communicating between professionals, as the basis for research, and for the design and planning of services. Flo Bellamy, in an online blog, described this in practice.[18] Flo reported that someone she knew '... said she was labelled as a personality disorder and experienced severe depression and suicidal ideation. She said no one understood what she meant when she said those words and everyone would go silent or change the subject. Another in the group asked, "What did you say *before* you had any experience of the mental health world?" to which she replied, "Well I said I felt like shit and that I wanted to kill myself." To which the other person said, "And did people understand that?" She had to admit that they did.'

It would be inappropriate to try to list every problem that it's possible to experience. But we can easily see how some of the diagnoses already mentioned could be replaced with more appropriate language. We understand what it means when someone is feeling low, has intrusive anxious thoughts or feels compelled to carry out certain behaviours such as checking things. We understand what attention problems are, what it means to hear voices, and so on. There should be no particular surprise that we can identify and define such specific phenomena. The Oxford English Dictionary defines the scientific method as: 'a method or procedure that has characterized natural science since the 17th century, consisting in systematic observation, measurement, and experiment, and the formulation, testing, and modification of hypotheses.' So scientists use operational (precise) definitions of relevant concepts. We develop hypotheses. And we collect data. We don't need to meet the challenge of a new technological alternative to diagnosis and the 'disease model'. We've had it since the 17th century.

Oddly and rather sadly, the diagnostic approach takes this rather strong position and then perverts it. The individual components, the 'symptoms', can each be identified with some rigour. But when they are combined into 'disorders' through the application of the rules for combining 'symptoms', the rigour is lost. We can reliably and validly identify 'auditory hallucinations', 'delusional beliefs' or 'thought disorder' (although it would be possible and preferable to use some less pejorative names). But that validity is lost when we try to identify 'schizophrenia'.

Reassuringly, the list of likely problems need not be particularly long. While there are estimated to be over 200 different psychiatric diagnoses, the number of individual problems is actually much smaller. That is not only counter-intuitive, it undermines a fundamental idea behind diagnosis – the idea that 'symptoms' cluster into 'disorders'. There is not (yet) an accepted or definitive list of problems – and there probably doesn't have to be such a list. If someone came with a problem which, as yet, nobody else had ever experienced, that doesn't strike me as too much of an issue – we simply respond appropriately to that unique challenge. I'm sure, for instance, that both the person reporting the problem, and the profession to whom they report it would be able to describe it in straightforward language. But there is good reason to suppose that a relatively short list of common problems would cover most people's experiences.

In 2009, a doctoral student, Gemma Parker, Simon Duff and I looked at the statistical validity of diagnoses using a statistical technique called smallest space analysis.[19] We found, like many others, that individual experiences did not cluster together as predicted by the disease-model diagnostic approach, but rather specific problems seemed to be distributed on a continuous basis. To perform this analysis however, Gemma first had to extract the specific problems or phenomena themselves. She identified only 65 different specific symptoms within DSM-IV (this was, of course, conducted before the revision of the franchise). More recently, a colleague of mine conducting her PhD studies – Kate Allsopp – conducted the same breakdown of constituent elements of ICD-10. She identified only 57 common problems.

In retrospect, it is quite simple to see how a relatively simple list of problems can generate a confusing plethora of diagnoses. Imagine a world in which people present with only three problems. If they were randomly distributed amongst the 57 possibilities, we could imagine 57x56x55 or 175,560 different combinations for each person. That is a huge number, but it also highlights how flexible a problem-list approach could be.

This helps to highlight important differences between a problem-list approach and a diagnostic approach. When I, or colleagues, recommend replacing diagnoses with simple problem-lists, people who are keen on diagnoses often suggest that they are essentially the same thing – that a set of diagnoses essentially *is* a list of problems. But there are many essential differences. Diagnoses are generated by combining symptoms with 'if–then' rules ('schizophrenia', for example, is diagnosed when a person has one of a number of possible combinations of individual problems: they hear voices and are frightened that people may do them harm, but have not recently experienced a bereavement, to give one of many possible combinations). A problem-list approach explicitly keeps these problems separate. Only a very small number of diagnoses have only one symptom. And 'symptoms' are essentially specific problems. There is an essential philosophical difference between identifying a problem and identifying a 'symptom'. In the latter case, the clear implication is that the 'symptom' is the result of an illness, and probably a biological illness at that. Perhaps the main reason that professionals feel the need to reduce any one person's complex plethora of problems to a single 'diagnosis' is to try and simplify things. But, while simplicity is an admirable goal, the mistake here is in attempting – as the Times editorial put it – to do the impossible *where definition is impossible*. Moreover, since a problem-list approach is inherently both simple and flexible (with 175,560 different ways of combining three choices of 57 problems), we already have workable alternatives to diagnosis.

## Planning, commissioning and audit

At present, much of healthcare is planned, audited and commissioned on the basis of diagnosis. The supposed reliance on diagnosis to plan and commission care is a mainstay of the arguments that diagnosis is necessary. However, it doesn't have to be that way. For individuals, as I shall explain below, individual care plans can be – and in fact frequently are – developed without recourse to diagnosis. And it simply isn't necessary for planning purposes either. I am constantly proud of the UK's National Health Service, a comprehensive system ensuring world-class healthcare available to all, free at the point of need and predicated on the principles of universal and equitable provision. Other nations are less fortunate, and still rely heavily on either commercial provision or on services funded through insurance. In these latter schemes, diagnosis is often important in gaining access to services, and services therefore suffer. In the UK, diagnostic information – incidence and prevalence – are important, but not of overwhelming significance. As we'll see in Chapter 8, services are currently commissioned on the basis of a wide range of parameters, in liaison with local authority social services through the joint Health and Wellbeing Boards. These parameters include prevalence statistics – which in turn rely on diagnosis – but are not dominated by them. This means that we can easily imagine a system for the commissioning of services that would not be predicated on diagnosis. In other settings – in education, in social services, in criminal justice services – we do not rely on diagnosis. That doesn't mean that such services are aimless or random. Instead, well-developed systems of service commissioning are in place, based upon the identification of problems and the evidence-base for available services.

We do, of course, need to know the extent of the problems that we have to address, and the scale of the response needed. We need to know how many psychological therapists, how many psychologists, how many psychiatrists to employ. We need to know what type of residential services to commission, and how many people will be needed to staff them. We need to know the extent of the problems; how many working days are lost each year to emotional problems, how many children are finding it difficult to attend to their school work (and who might need the help of educational psychologists). Commissioners and planners of services need answers to questions that are unrelated to diagnosis. They need to know how many people experience certain problems, the economic costs associated with those problems, and the recommended interventions. It is a perfectly valid question to ask how many employment advisors are needed in our mental health services, but knowing how many people have a certain diagnosis doesn't tell us that. Once again, we need information about specific problems, specific needs and specific circumstances, not diagnoses, to plan for care.

## Psychosocial formulations

In order to understand and explain people's experiences, and in order to plan services, we need to do a little more than simply make a list of problems (even if we do assess the severity of those problems on continua or dimensions). This is, of course, recognised by medical psychiatrists, who equally understand that people – patients – need to be offered more than a mere diagnosis. For clinical psychologists, this means developing psychological 'formulations'. It is via these formulations that we can recognise the fact that psychosocial factors such as poverty, unemployment and trauma are the most well-established causes of psychological distress[20] although, of course, we must also acknowledge that other factors – for example, genetic and developmental – may influence the way in which each individual reacts to challenges.

Psychological formulations are attempts to describe why people are experiencing difficulties and what might help, based on psychosocial principles and with reference to psychological theories. Formulations take as their starting point a problem that the person describes, rather than a diagnosis or a professional's opinion. So a well-founded formulation would address such problems as low mood and lack of motivation, hearing voices, problems functioning at work, paranoia etc. That would be different than, for example, formulations about 'schizophrenia', which would generally fail, for the reasons outlined here.

Clinical psychologists therefore work with their clients, and are informed by psychological science, to develop hypotheses about what might have led to the development of these problems and, consequently, theories about what might be helpful. Clearly, the more precise information we have about the exact problems for which the person is seeking help, the events and circumstances of their lives, as well as how they have responded and what things they have done to try to help, the better the formulation will be. Because all these issues are highly personal, formulations are necessarily very individual, tailored for each person and their specific problems.

Many professions rightly emphasise the importance of formulations. Those developed by psychologists (as one would expect) place particular emphasis on psychological processes to explain and account for the problems. That means a focus on the way that people make sense of their world. In the words of the Health and Care Professions Council (the regulatory body for clinical psychologists in the UK), clinical psychologists must ' … understand psychological models related to how biological, sociological and circumstantial or life-event related factors impinge on psychological processes to affect psychological well-being … '.

## This matters

This is not just an academic issue. 'Diagnoses' send an inappropriate message about the nature of mental health problems. It is inappropriate to suggest that a 'disease' called 'depression' is responsible for the low mood someone is experiencing. It is inappropriate philosophically, because it confuses a label with an explanation. It doesn't help to say that the label that we give to the experience of low mood is the cause of the low mood. It doesn't help us understand why a person is hearing voices to suggest that the cause of the voices is a disorder called 'schizophrenia'. 'Schizophrenia' is again merely a label we give to a variety of problems, including hallucinations. This is inappropriate because it's lazy thinking, and it's inappropriate because it pretends to offer an explanation, but fails so to do. This is probably most worrying when parents need to understand why their child has problems with attention or emotion regulation. To say: '...he is having problems concentrating at school because he has ADHD...' is so circular, so misleading, that it is genuinely counter-productive.

I have previously mentioned how diagnoses, in the area of mental health, can also have very serious implications for people. Diagnosis is stigmatising, but the labels can also have significant practical consequences for people. I have had personal experience, through my professional activity, of people whose careers have been threatened by psychiatric diagnoses offered during childhood. In the majority of cases, these diagnoses had been used speculatively – with possible diagnoses recorded in medical records without a great deal of confidence in their accuracy or the likely consequences. In most cases, medication was either recommended or prescribed, but the clients rarely took the medication regularly. However, later in their lives, when applying for responsible jobs, the previous 'psychiatric diagnoses' tended to have very serious consequences – it is sometimes very bad news, in a competitive and risk-averse world, to have 'mental illness' in your medical history. Writer Fay Thomas, 'diagnosed' with bipolar disorder, has argued eloquently that we should treat psychiatric diagnoses as potentially defamatory.[21]

But perhaps the most important negative consequence of a psychiatric diagnosis is what happens next. After we have been diagnosed with a 'mental disorder', it's a near-certainty that we'll be prescribed medication. The diagnosis of depression is intimately associated with the prescription of 'antidepressants'. The diagnosis of 'ADHD' leads inexorably to a prescription for Ritalin. The diagnosis of 'schizophrenia' leads to a prescription for 'antipsychotic' medication. And I absolutely don't think drugs are the answer.

# 3
# The Drugs Don't Work... So Offer Real Solutions

*We should sharply reduce our reliance on medication to address emotional distress. Medication should be used sparingly and in response to specific problems. Our current heavy reliance on psychiatric medication is based on flawed logic. Many chemicals are known to affect our mood and thinking, and there is no clear evidence that psychiatric medication is correcting underlying biochemical abnormalities. Psychiatric medication, taken long-term, also appears to have some very distressing adverse effects. Rather than seeing mental health as a biological or medical issue and assuming that medication will 'cure' non-existent underlying 'illnesses', medication instead should be used sparingly and in response to specific problems. In practice, this means adopting Dr Joanna Moncrieff's 'drug-based' approach in contrast to the more common 'disease-based' approach.*

Mental health care is naturally an issue of political significance. A frequently quoted figure suggests that one in four of us are likely to experience significant mental health difficulties at some point in our lives. There are reasons to question this figure since statistics like these often rely on diagnoses – counting the number of people who meet the criteria for a mental health diagnosis. It follows that, if we are sceptical of diagnoses, we should be sceptical of these figures. But what is clear is that the numbers of us affected are huge. According to the World Health Organization, poor mental health is the single greatest cause of disability worldwide,[1] and in England alone, the costs of poor mental health are estimated at £105 billion per year.[2] So it is right and proper that politicians take an interest in these matters.

There was a landmark debate recently in the UK House of Commons. Several MPs took the opportunity to speak movingly of their own psychological problems…and to call for radical new approaches in our thinking. British MPs are not the only politicians to be open about mental health issues. The Norwegian Prime Minister, Kjell Magne Bondevik, announced in 1998 that he was stepping away from his post, saying that he was depressed. For three weeks, his deputy took over, until Bondevik returned. More remarkably, Bondevik's government lost a motion of 'no confidence' in 2000 and lost power for about 18 months. Bondevik, however, led his party in the next general election, and returned to power, as Prime Minister, to lead a successful coalition government. It's worth repeating that. After discussing his depression openly, and after relinquishing the role of Prime Minister as a result, Bondevik won a general election and returned with a more secure public mandate.

In the UK House of Commons, Charles Walker MP memorably and equally bravely used the debate to discuss his own battles with persistent obsessive thoughts. Like many other people in his situation, he also discussed the most common form of help offered to people – medication:

> Let us look at these, more startling statistics. In 2009, the NHS issued 39.1 million prescriptions for anti-depressants – there was a big jump during the financial crisis, towards the end of the last decade. That figure represented a 95% increase on the decade, from the 20.2 million prescriptions issued in 1998. Were all of those 40 million prescriptions necessary? Of course they were not.[3]

I agree. I also fail to accept that these 40 million prescriptions for anti-depressants are necessary. With fewer than 60 million people of working age in the UK, this is a simply astonishing number (even if we accept that very many of these prescriptions are never given to pharmacists, let alone the actual medication taken). And it's also the wrong kind of help.

Charles Walker MP expressed this very clearly:

> We can talk about medical solutions to mental health problems, and of course medicine has a part to play. In reality, however, society has the biggest part to play. This is society's problem.

His fellow Member of Parliament, James Morris MP, made a similar point:

> …we must also examine whether our approach to tackling the problem is fit and appropriate for the 21st century. Our approach to

mental illness over a number of decades has been based on what I would call the psychiatric model. The model has medicalised mental illness and treated it as something to be dealt with using drug-based therapies.

As we have seen earlier, Charles Walker and James Morris are correct. These are serious problems. But they are serious social problems. And they should be addressed with social solutions.

This level of prescription also comes at an astonishing cost. It has been estimated[4] that we spend around £800 million per year in the UK on psychiatric drugs. The prescription of antidepressant medication alone costs the UK National Health Service over £200 million per year. We spend £44 million on stimulants and other drugs prescribed to children for the 'treatment' of 'ADHD' or 'Attention Deficit Hyperactivity Disorder'. I agree with Charles Walker; a very large proportion (at least) of this spending is probably wasted. Although some people find medication helpful, I believe that we need to balance the positive effects of taking medication – which are almost certainly short-lived in most instances – against their adverse effects.

## A pill to take away your sadness

I am a clinical psychologist. I believe I have a good working knowledge of the evidence-base for the effectiveness of pharmacological interventions and I think I have some understanding of the hypothesised biological mechanisms. But I do rely on the expertise of my colleagues with more specialist skills, experience, knowledge and qualifications. One unequivocal expert is Dr Joanna Moncrieff, to whom I turn for systematic and intelligent reviews of the literature. In her books 'The Myth of the Chemical Cure' and 'The Bitterest Pills',[5] and online[6] Jo reviews a great deal of the evidence about the extent to which psychiatric drugs are effective in helping people, and discusses the related issue of whether they are 'treating illnesses' in any meaningful sense.

Because antidepressants are prescribed so frequently, it seems likely that at least some people think they 'work'. And – at least in the UK and most other post-industrial democracies – clinicians are helped to make appropriate decisions about prescription through complicated processes that involve expert panels making recommendations on the basis of systematic reviews of published scientific evidence. Those processes lead to such useful tools as the clinical guidelines issued by the National Institute for Health and Care Excellence or NICE. These guidelines – and therefore the systematic reviews on which they are based – conclude that antidepressants 'work'. In Joanna Moncrieff's words: 'the general feeling seems to be that although they are being overused and may have some unpleasant side-effects, they certainly "work", at least in some people'.[7]

Perhaps the first thing to say – because often this striking point is not mentioned – is that we know that a huge range of chemicals affect our perceptions, moods and thoughts. Although it might be unwise, there are vanishingly few people who never ingest psychoactive substances. Across the world, in most cultures, people drink alcohol (which affects their brain chemistry), chew khat (ditto), smoke nicotine-delivering ciga-rettes, and drink coffee (which has well-recognised effects on the brain, as well as on the digestive system). Laws and social rules differ across the world, but there are enormous markets for illegal drugs – cannabis, ecstasy, heroin, cocaine, LSD etc. I don't advocate taking such street or recreational drugs (although I'm not very keen on legal prohibition or the 'war on drugs', either). The essential point is that many chemicals of many kinds – foods, illegal and legal drugs – change our thoughts, perceptions and moods. The three groups of drugs we are discussing here – recreational street drugs, commonplace drugs such as alcohol and caffeine, and doctor-prescribed medication – all follow the basic laws of biochemistry. The medication prescribed in response to mental distress is specifically designed to alter our mood. So, in that context, it would be foolish to expect 'antidepressants', 'antipsychotics' or other psychiatric drugs to have no discernible effects. Of course they'll affect our moods. That's not surprising. But – and this is the important point – that's rather different from thinking that 'antidepressants' specifically target under-lying biological abnormalities responsible for an illness – depression – and therefore can be regarded as treatments for that condition.

The conventional approach to testing the effectiveness of medica-tion and other therapies is to conduct a 'randomised controlled trial' or RCT. I've been involved in a few. Clinical recommendations – such as NICE guidelines – are typically based on systematic reviews of many such RCTs. And systematic reviews of the effectiveness of antidepres-sants[8] suggest that, on average, people taking antidepressants see their scores on a mood rating scale improve a little more than people who are taking a placebo or nothing. The difference in improvement – the degree to which antidepressants out-perform placebos – is enough to establish beyond statistical chance that the medication has some kind of effect. It's worth saying that this degree of change is typically about the same as that offered by psychological therapies such as CBT (cognitive behavioural therapy). And it's also important to note that, typically, both the people given the antidepressants (or CBT) *and* the people given the placebo *both* see their low mood ease over time. There are many reasons for this, including the fact that people typically seek help when their mood is low, and therefore their mood is likely to improve over time – fortunately not many of us remain depressed for long periods.

More importantly, we need to understand what this means in practice. Again, all these caveats apply equally to trials of psychological therapies. But what counts as 'effective' in the language of such clinical trials may not be quite what we expect. First, it only means that the degree to which antidepressants out-perform the placebo is 'statistically significant'. That is, the difference is relatively unlikely to be due to chance. That doesn't mean it's necessarily a large difference. NICE guidelines recommend the use of antidepressants on the basis that many studies have found such differences, rather than because antidepressants are dramatically effective. In addition, many scientists and academics are concerned[9] that drugs companies and researchers routinely fail to publish negative results (meaning that only the positive results see the light of day).

In nearly all such trials, outcome is assessed on the basis of scores on questionnaire measures of low mood. In many senses, that's reasonable. Since problems such as low mood lie on continua – some people feel desperately low, some people are quite miserable, others are broadly happy – it is better to measure the degree of somebody's low mood than to ask whether they are or are not experiencing 'depression'. And since only the person themselves can really say what they are experiencing, 'self-report' questionnaires are appropriate ways to measure these things. But there is an issue when we look at what counts as 'improvement'. Randomised controlled trials are powerful ways of discovering differences between two groups, but whilst there might be an average difference between the groups, there is usually still a very great deal of overlap. In a typical trial, it is possible for there to be a difference between two groups (for instance, those people taking antidepressants versus those taking placebos) of only two points on a questionnaire with a maximum score of 54. And the questionnaires used to assess low mood cover quite a wide range of problems. Typically, people will be asked about their mood, their motivation, their ability to enjoy life, their sleeping, their appetite, and their self-esteem. Although obviously any improvement in scores is good, improvements of two or three points on these scales could well reflect improved motivation, better sleep or better appetite rather than an improvement in mood itself. These are effects that could well be related to medication. But they don't necessarily represent a 'cure' for 'depression'.

A few years ago I was involved in a small study that looked at the effects of different clothing on our mood.[10] It was a pretty straightforward study; we asked people to wear outfits they liked and also ones they didn't and asked them about their moods – using the same kinds of questionnaires used in measuring the outcome of trials of antidepressants. Unsurprisingly, the people felt better – happier and more confident – wearing outfits that they preferred. Unsurprisingly, these differences weren't huge...but they were about the magnitude of the differences usually reported for antidepressants. When we've had good news, our mood lifts a little. When we receive a compliment, our mood lifts a little. When we wear clothes we like, our mood lifts a little. When I have a cup of coffee (I'm not going to speak for anybody else here), I feel my mood lift a little. And when people take antidepressants, on average, their mood appears to lift...a little.

## Are antidepressants 'antidepressants', or just drugs?

Joanna Moncrieff points out several problems with a 'disease model' of drug action – the assumption (on the basis of their name, perhaps) that psychiatric medication offers 'cures' for 'illnesses'. The two previous chapters contained detailed discussions of the inadequacies of the twin concepts of the biomedical disease model of mental health problems, and psychiatric diagnosis. It is obvious that people can become depressed. I have no doubt that 'depression' exists as a phenomenon. But I don't believe it is right to suggest that depression exists as an illness. As I outlined in Chapter 2, there are very many understandable reasons why people can become demoralised, unhappy and pessimistic. So people obviously have periods of very low mood. They very obviously become depressed. We have a clear moral imperative to offer help. But that isn't the same thing as saying that there exists an 'illness' that requires a 'treatment'.

Antidepressants are chemicals that affect the functioning of the brain. Older antidepressants tended to be rather sedating – in other words, they made people feel tired and slowed down. This was, of course, rather unpleasant, and often dangerous. More modern antidepressants have been chosen or designed, very carefully in some cases, to affect our moods, but to avoid these sedating effects. They can, still, make people drowsy or lethargic. They can sometimes induce a sense of indifference, which for some people, helpfully takes the edge off their feelings of despair, but which others find unpleasant or even distressing. They can have other effects such as sexual dysfunction or feelings of agitation.

These are, just as with street drugs, the chemical effects of the medication on the functioning of the brain. Some people may find the effects helpful. If you are feeling lethargic, a drug that improves your alertness may be helpful. Many people who are in a state of distress experience unpleasant intrusive thoughts, and sometimes ruminate on their problems. In that case, a sense of emotional detachment, brought about by a psychiatric drug, may be helpful. People who are depressed, especially if they are also anxious, may find that a reduction in anxiety and a slight sedative effect is calming and helps sleep. All these changes – which I would argue are recognisable and understandable effects of drugs, whether prescribed or recreational – may be negative or positive. They may well lead to changes on rating scales designed to assess the severity of a depressed mood. But it seems difficult to argue that these medication-induced changes in emotional states represent genuine therapeutic gains. They are real and in a sense genuine; but they are what they are – the understandable effects of psychoactive chemicals.

There is no good evidence that these chemicals are correcting any underlying biological mechanism. There is a danger that people are being subtly misled about the effects of medication. People are often under the impression that the medication is putting right some underlying abnormality, whereas it would be much more honest to outline the general psychoactive and physical effects of the medication. Then people could weigh up any possible benefits against possible adverse effects, and decide themselves whether or not these effects might be useful. There are many chemicals that affect our emotions, perceptions, thought and behaviour. People swallow or smoke these chemicals for understandable reasons, and the chemicals – the drugs – have a range of effects, both good and bad. That's a long way short of a 'treatment' for an 'illness'.

Unfortunately, the possible positive effects of psychiatric medication come with a cost. Antidepressant drugs have some unpleasant adverse effects, too. Some of the newer 'selective serotonin reuptake inhibitors' or SSRIs can lead to sexual dysfunction and loss of libido, which may be related to the phenomenon of emotional indifference that some people experience. There have been very distressing reports of people having intrusive suicidal thoughts, and some researchers believe that antidepressants are associated with an increased risk of suicide, especially in young people. This may be related to the tendency for antidepressants – unsurprisingly – to make people more motivated and impulsive, which might be good in some ways but also somewhat risky in someone who is depressed. And many people report having severe and prolonged withdrawal reactions (for further discussion of all these problems, see Jo Moncrieff's 'The Myth of the Chemical Cure'[11]).

Representatives of pharmaceutical companies, and some psychiatrists, stress that antidepressants 'aren't addictive'. This seems very important – people are naturally worried about the addictive power of cigarettes, street drugs and some older forms of psychiatric medication such as the benzodiazepines (valium, etc.). It's reassuring for people contemplating taking prescribed antidepressants to know that they 'aren't addictive'. It does seem odd, and a strange use of language, however. Addiction is surprisingly difficult to define, but best refers to a person's dependence on something (in this case drugs) to be able to function normally. It's quite common to hear representatives of pharmaceutical companies comment that 'antidepressants aren't addictive', but then qualify this by saying 'but people can experience a recurrence of their depressive symptoms when they stop taking the drugs'. Which sounds very similar to needing the drugs to function normally. In fact … isn't that the main selling point of the medication?

The research tells me that antidepressant medication might be slightly better than a placebo at raising people's mood. That's not in itself something to be sniffed at. But the positive effects certainly come with some rather nasty side-effects. The positive effects aren't dramatic, and they don't appear to represent a 'cure'. Researchers haven't been able to identify abnormal biological pathways that are targeted by the antidepressants, and in that context, the discovery of some chemicals that alter brain chemistry to make people feel a little better is hardly ground-breaking science.

## A pill to take away your madness

The potential benefits of taking antidepressants seem underwhelming when set against their costs. A similar but subtly different argument applies to long-term so-called 'antipsychotic' medication. There are some benefits for people in acute distress, and with particular problems, from taking antipsychotic drugs. But taken longer term, these drugs have serious, life-changing adverse effects. These negative effects, sometimes euphemistically called 'side-effects', can include a condition that resembles Parkinson's disease – with shaking, muscular rigidity and problems with walking and movement – and even reduced brain size in people who have been taking 'antipsychotic' medication for a long time. Because they affect various physical systems, such as our heart, liver and kidneys, as well as our brains, and because one of the common adverse effects is a significant gain in weight (itself physically dangerous), these drugs can have a significant impact on our health.

Dr Joanna Moncrieff reports on her blog a story of a woman who was very distressed by frightening psychotic experiences.[12] The woman was scared that she had a gadget implanted in her body and that she was being watched and manipulated by malignant forces. Psychotic experiences like this are surprisingly common, and obviously very distressing for the person involved. Dr Moncrieff reports how, as we might expect, the young woman began taking an antipsychotic drug. As is common, Joanna reports that as the dose was gradually increased the young woman 'became increasingly quiet, subdued, emotionless, expressionless and physically sluggish'. Dr Moncrieff contrasts the medical consensus – that the young woman was 'better' – with her own perspective – that the young woman's life 'seemed empty and lifeless...although admittedly less distressed'.

To me, this sums up both my own experience of observing people taking antipsychotic drugs and the scientific consensus. These powerful drugs are effective at helping people calm down and can sometimes reduce distress, but can hardly be considered cures. They have very clear effects on people, and those effects can be helpful. But they don't target biological abnormalities specific to psychosis, and don't return people to 'normal'. They just have the kinds of effects that psychoactive drugs are recognised to have.

I need to be clear here. I understand that antipsychotic drugs can be very helpful. In acute emergencies (especially, perhaps, when people are very agitated), antipsychotic medication can be enormously helpful and even life-saving. Decisions about medication are, or certainly should be, individual issues. Blanket advice one way or another would be foolish. But it does appear that antipsychotic medication can be helpful in suppressing acute psychotic symptoms. And it's important to recognise that many people experience highly distressing psychotic phenomena for years, either on an on-going or a recurrent basis. Again, that means that for some people, as Jo Moncrieff puts it: 'life on long-term drug treatment, even with all its drawbacks, might be preferable to life without it'.[12]

There is a great deal of debate about the changes that have taken place in inpatient psychiatric care over the past six decades, and particularly about the reasons for the dramatic reduction in the number of in-patient residents in psychiatric hospitals. One line of argument suggests that this was the result of profound changes both in society and in nursing practices. The most widely-accepted opinion is that the development of chlorpromazine in the 1950's allowed, for the first time, many thousands of people to achieve some form of relief from their distress. It's clear that many people in the early decades of the 20th century, and before, could spend many years of their lives in extreme distress. It would be stupid and cruel to deny people such help.

But we also need to be clear what the effects of these drugs are, and whether they are either 'cures' or, in fact, 'antipsychotics'. That is, do they target an underlying biological abnormality, return a person to a state of normality and substantially remove the problems? We might also add: do they prevent relapse? It seems clear, and seems to have been clear back in the 1950s, that antipsychotic drugs such as chlorpromazine numb people's emotions. These can reduce emotional distress (so can, I repeat, be a good thing), but is not quite the same thing as reducing psychosis. People who are convinced that others mean them harm (with 'paranoid delusions', in psychiatric language), and who are very frightened that they are in imminent danger, will often find their fears much less preoccupying and distressing if they take chlorpromazine.[13] That sounds a lot like the effects of opioid street drugs like heroin.

A study of the recent history of psychiatry also tells us that the ways in which medication has been used, and discussed, have changed over time. Initially, psychiatrists appeared to use medication pragmatically to help reduce distress and agitation, and acknowledged its direct effects (some psychiatrists quite overtly described them as damaging the brain). But over time, psychiatrists began to think of drugs as 'treatments' for underlying conditions. The drugs shifted from being practical short-term solutions to long-term or prophylactic preventative remedies. Current clinical guidelines recommend long-term treatment with antipsychotic medication for people who have been given the diagnosis of 'schizophrenia'.[14] Those recommendations parallel the growing assumption that the antipsychotic drugs are sophisticated treatments, specifically designed to correct an underlying biological abnormality that causes their problems.

It seems clear that 'antipsychotic' medication is helpful for some people, especially in the short term and if they are very distressed. It seems much less clear that antipsychotic medication prevents relapse. This, again, needs to be considered very carefully. Some people have on-going problems, and may find that medication which helps to lessen their distress is useful for long periods. But that isn't quite the basis on which antipsychotic medication is often recommended, namely that it prevents a 'relapse' – a return of the psychotic experiences. That seems a much less certain prospect.

The use of antipsychotic medication on a long-term basis (daily or even injected as a 'depot') is so ubiquitous that it is quite difficult to find comparisons between groups of people who have, and have not, taken the drugs for long periods of time. These kinds of comparisons are also difficult because the medications are very powerful, so that when people stop taking their drugs (especially without expert medical advice), they often experience profound and distressing withdrawal effects, which can either resemble or induce the return of their previous psychotic experiences. However the emerging evidence, summarised in books by Richard Bentall, Robert Whitaker and Jo Moncrieff[15] strongly suggests that for most people the long-term benefits of antipsychotic medication are significantly outweighed by their profound adverse effects. And it looks very much as if the levels of psychosis, and 'relapse' rates, are no higher in people who live medication-free lives than in people who take antipsychotic medication on a long-term basis. In other words, these drugs don't appear to prevent relapse. And, because these drugs have very profound side-effects, those people who take the medication on a long-term basis often experience significant physical health problems, as well as emotional blunting, sedation and suppression of creativity and imagination. Many wise and intelligent psychiatrists therefore conclude, as Joanna Moncrieff has done, that 'these are not innocuous drugs, and people should be given the opportunity to see if they can manage without them, both during an acute psychotic episode and after recovery from one' and that 'if you reduce people's antipsychotics in a gradual and supported manner, people are better off in the long-term. Some will manage to stop their antipsychotics completely and do well, and overall people will not suffer higher levels of symptoms or relapses than if they had stayed on their original level of medication.'

It is worth pointing out that many of these concerns also apply to medication used to 'treat' so-called 'bipolar disorder'. People experience episodes of depression, and some people experience episodes of mania (feeling very agitated or 'high', sometimes leading to actions you later regret such as running up large bills) or hypomania (the same but to a slightly lesser degree). Let's leave aside for a moment the issue of whether this diagnosis is valid or helpful, except to say that in my view it adds nothing to label a tendency to experience extreme moods 'bipolar disorder'.[16] Manic episodes can be distressing and dangerous, and people who experience a manic episode once are highly likely to experience another one. That does demand a response. Antipsychotic medication can be helpful as an immediate or emergency response, but there is much less evidence for the effectiveness of the two main medications that are often used to prevent 'relapse'.[17] Because recurrent episodes of mania and depression can be disabling, there is real pressure to prescribe drugs that can be effective not only in an acute episode, but as prophylaxis – that is, to reduce the likelihood of future episodes. Lithium (a so-called 'mood stabiliser' is the most commonly-used medication, but long-term antipsychotics are also commonly prescribed. And here too there are major doubts as to their effectiveness. Just as with psychosis, there is precious little evidence that the medication is targeting any underlying biological abnormalities.

## So why do we take them?

A recent editorial in the British Medical Journal[18] discussed this very issue. The statistics are frightening. The UK trend is replicated across the developed world, with a doubling in the number of antidepressants over the past 10 years.[19] According to the US National Center for Health Statistics, in 2011, 11% of Americans aged 12 and over were taking antidepressants. One partial explanation for this amazing statistic may be a massive level of over-diagnosis. As I reported in the previous chapter, diagnostic criteria are loose and vague, and include a range of common and normal experiences. It has been suggested that only 38% of people whom clinicians diagnose with 'depression' would actually meet standard diagnostic criteria.[20] I have some problems with this analysis – I don't regard depression as a valid concept but merely a label that should be reserved for people with more serious difficulties, and I believe it is simply wrong to use such disease metaphors for normal human responses to difficult circumstances. Nevertheless, it is clear that very many people are receiving these damaging labels, and, therefore, receiving prescriptions for these non-existent illnesses.

The international pharmaceutical companies are not innocent, either. Massive and well-funded marketing efforts are employed to sell drugs to prescribing physicians or (where the nation's legislation allows it) direct to the consumer. In his excellent book 'Cracked: Why Psychiatry Is Doing More Harm Than Good',[21] James Davies describes the effort that pharmaceutical companies expend and the lengths to which they go in order to convince people to consume their products. These range from excessive promotion of positive findings through to the frankly immoral and deliberate hiding of negative ones. This is important – if industry-sponsored drug trials with negative findings (in other words, where the drugs are not shown to be successful) are suppressed, the only journal articles that are available for review are the positive ones. In consequence, the drugs appear much more effective than they really are. Researchers – particularly, but not exclusively, academic psychiatrists – are also implicated. Some appear to be very well remunerated for promoting drugs companies' products. Between 2000 and 2007, the psychiatrist Professor Charles Nemeroff received $2.8 million (personally) from drugs companies while supposedly acting as an impartial scientist overseeing trials of the drugs manufactured by the companies remunerating him. Similarly, Dr Joseph Biederman was dubbed the 'King of Ritalin' after receiving $1.6 million in consultancy fees from drugs companies.

But perhaps the most important marketing technique is to suggest that the human distress that triggers a desire to offer help is an 'illness'. Because while the understandable distress that follows the loss of a loved one triggers empathy, a listening ear and practical help, the diagnosis of a 'major depressive episode' is likely to lead to a prescription for antidepressant medication.

The well-known mouthwash, Listerine, was originally developed as a surgical antiseptic. Its main active ingredients are essential oils and alcohol. The product was subsequently sold as a floor-cleaning product and (slightly bizarrely) as a cure for gonorrhoea. The product became highly profitable, however, in the 1920's, when it was marketed as a cure for 'halitosis'. We all know that people can occasionally have bad breath. And so it makes sense to offer products that can address this problem. The genius of the Listerine marketing strategy was to develop the quasi-medical concept of halitosis – a problem for which Listerine was the solution. This happens across mental health. People occasionally experience low mood – often in response to negative life events. But 'depression' is an illness that (so the logic goes) requires the prescription of anti-depressant medication. People occasionally have very distressing psychotic experiences – often in response to childhood trauma. But 'schizophrenia' is an illness that (the argument goes) requires the prescription of antipsychotic medication. Manic episodes can be a major threat to someone's well-being, and it would be very sensible both to consider what medication might be helpful when they happen, and also to learn how to identify the early warning signs of episodes and help to avoid them. But 'bipolar disorder' is an illness that (it is argued) requires the prescription of prophylactic medication. Children occasionally have problems paying attention in class. But 'Attention Deficit Hyperactivity Disorder or ADHD' is an illness (so the logic goes) that requires the prescription of stimulants such as Ritalin.

A good example of this phenomenon is the history of Wellbutrin, a brand name for the drug bupropion. Bupropion appears to have its effect on the central nervous system by interacting with dopamine receptors, and it clearly has effects. It is considered moderately dangerous in overdose, when it leads to hallucinations, delusions, vomiting, aggressive behaviour and seizures and has been associated with deaths. The side-effects are, genuinely, too many to list here. On the (perhaps) more positive front, bupropion has been recommended as an appropriate treatment for: smoking cessation, 'seasonal affective disorder', 'attention deficit hyperactivity disorder' or ADHD, sexual dysfunction, obesity (or more properly, appetite suppression), and inflammatory bowel disease. It is quite widely used as an antidepressant. So far, Wellbutrin or bupropion looks much like any other psychiatric drug – it has central nervous system effects, but can't in all honesty be said to be a specific treatment for a specific illness by targeting a specific biological pathology. Wellbutrin is particularly interesting because it looks very much like a product in need of an illness for which it is the treatment. And the recent decision to remove bereavement as an exclusion criterion for the diagnosis of depression may offer that opportunity. That is, there have been hints that some psychiatrists are attempting to demonstrate that Wellbutrin is an effective treatment for depression associated with bereavement.[22] This is extraordinary ... find a drug that struggles to find a market, re-label a normal human response to a sad but commonplace event as a symptom of an 'illness', and then prescribe the product as a treatment for that 'illness'.

## Drugs are drugs

Dr Joanna Moncrieff raised some intriguing questions in a recent blog. 'Using psychoactive substances to cope with negative emotions is a longstanding human response, but also one that is fraught with difficulty. Although drug-induced effects may bring temporary relief, they may also hamper people from finding more lasting solutions to their problems. If people do want to go down this route, however, there seems no reason to restrict the repertoire to drugs currently called "antidepressants". This raises all sorts of thorny questions, of course, about why some psychoactive drugs are legal and others illegal, about what sort of drug use society approves of and what it doesn't, and why the legal dispensation of many drugs is restricted to doctors.'[23]

I think Jo is raising some fascinating but difficult points here. There are a vast number of different chemicals that people ingest to alter their mood, perceptions or thought processes. There is also institutionalised hypocrisy. At one extreme, we have strict laws controlling the possession, sale and use of recreational street drugs, even a 'war' on drugs. At the other extreme, clinicians can use the Mental Health Act (or similar laws in other jurisdictions) to compel patients to adhere to treatment plans – which almost invariably mean prescriptions for medication. The use of chemicals to change your perceptions and mood seems simultaneously to be illegal and compulsory.

There are differences between different drugs. Crack cocaine is a highly addictive, therefore highly dangerous drug that acts, biologically, to increase levels of the neurotransmitters serotonin, norepinephrine and dopamine. These increased levels affect nerve functioning and make us feel good, but of course the drug also has other, harmful, consequences. The anti-depressant medication fluoxetine (Prozac) and related drugs known as SSRIs, 'selective serotonin reuptake inhibitors' – by definition – inhibit the reuptake of serotonin, but are designed to be more 'selective'. In practice, the different chemicals are all different; their detailed molecular structures affect their mode of action. Psychiatric medication and street drugs can both stimulate the production or release of neurotransmitters, and can block the reuptake of those neurotransmitters. The drugs can be specific (focussing on one neurotransmitter) or much more broad-spectrum in their effects. The time they take to work and then wear off can differ. They may also differ in the ways in which they stimulate the brain to respond – by producing more or less of the neurotransmitters, altering the sensitivity of neurotransmitter receptors, or even affecting the number of synapses (connections between nerve cells).

This means that the drugs – street recreational drugs or prescribed drugs – are all different. That could, at a stretch, justify an argument that some chemical formulations may be less harmful, and more closely tailored to the chemical effects that are desired than others. It could certainly mean that some drugs are more addictive than others – crack cocaine is notoriously addictive. Some psychoactive chemicals encourage further use because they have euphoric or other pleasurable effects, some because they reduce unpleasant emotions, and others because stopping taking them has negative consequences – withdrawal effects. It definitely means that we should choose our drugs with care (if you spend time talking to regular users of street drugs, or watch 'Breaking Bad', you learn that they are very knowledgeable about the effects of, and modes of action of, these products). But a drug is a drug is a drug. I'll give two quick examples: Ritalin, prescribed for children who have difficulty maintaining their attention in school, and ketamine, a veterinary tranquiliser. Both are stimulant drugs related to amphetamine. When people take amphetamine (an illegal recreational drug) they find it easier to concentrate, stay awake and work. That is true for all of us, not just children who have received the label of 'ADHD'. I'm not advocating the use of recreational amphetamines; but then I'm not advocating the prescription of stimulants to children with the diagnosis of 'ADHD'. Ketamine is a 'prescription only drug' in the UK, which means it is illegal to possess ketamine without a prescription. Ketamine is similarly illegal in many other countries. At the same time, ketamine is widely used as an antidepressant. It is claimed that ketamine can have an antidepressant effect within two hours ... which is presumably why it is popular as a recreational drug. Again, I'm not advocating the use of ketamine, either recreationally or by prescription.

These drugs have powerful effects on our brains. All such drugs have powerful effects on our brains. But it is difficult to make coherent distinctions between 'recreational' and 'prescription' drugs. We should exercise great care and caution over the choice whether or not to ingest such powerful chemicals. We need to understand the differences between the different drugs. We should probably take expert medical advice, from a professional who knows their subject well. But we shouldn't buy into the marketing myth that some chemicals are 'cures' for well-defined 'illnesses'.

## Stop pushing the drugs ... and offer real alternatives

The message from all of this is that we should be much more clear-sighted – more cynical, perhaps – more cautious and more sparing in our use of psychiatric drugs. In practical terms, we should aim for a massive reduction in the level of psychiatric prescription. There should be many fewer prescriptions, at lower doses, for much shorter periods. In essence, we should adopt Joanna Moncrieff's advice. We should respond to people's symptoms, rather than make the mistake that we're treating illnesses that can be identified by diagnosis. We should listen to the people's own experiences of how medication has and hasn't worked for them, or how it's working for them now, and use that as the basis of our prescribing. Perhaps most importantly, in the vast majority of cases we should use psychiatric medication in the very short term only.

This more pragmatic approach should see any use of psychiatric medication as part of a 'psychobiosocial model', where we at least attempt to understand why a person is distressed and how medication could act as a short-term adjunct to other forms of psychosocial care. This would echo

Joanna Moncrieff's 'drug-centred, not disease-centred' model, moving away from the myth that ingesting these chemicals in some sense 'cures' 'illnesses'. That would result, in practice, in a substantial reduction in the use of medication. We would see fewer prescriptions, for lower doses of medication, taken over shorter periods. To put some figures on it: we should aim immediately to reverse the doubling of prescriptions that has happened over the past decade – that is, halve the number of new psychiatric prescriptions immediately. A more reasonable medium-term aim would be to reduce the number of prescriptions to no more than 10% of their current levels. That, of course, would save the UK around £720 million per year in the costs of the drugs. It would save many thousands, even, millions, of people from the harm these drugs do to our bodies.

That, of course, would mean a profound change in the role of psychiatrists. At present, a large part of the role of the psychiatrist involves the 'diagnosis' of mental disorders and the prescription of medication. While the suggested vision for the future that I'm presenting here clearly does not exclude a medical element, it equally clearly suggests that medical colleagues need to adopt a different and more integrated role. If we accept a 'psychobiosocial' model for mental health care, and agree that medical advice concerning the use of psychiatric medication should be based on a pragmatic or 'drug-based' model, then it follows that community mental health teams would have a different relationship with medication and with the medical practitioners who bring expertise in its use.

Accepting a 'drug-based' approach to the prescription of psychiatric medication would not only see a substantial reduction in prescription, a focus on symptomatic relief rather than 'cure', and short-term rather than prophylactic prescription, but it would also see a shift of responsibility from secondary-care psychiatrists based in mental health trusts to GPs attached to community teams. The rationale for this is somewhat counter-factual. If psychiatric drugs were best thought of as highly specialist treatments that targeted discrete, diagnosable, illnesses then it would be perfectly appropriate to base policy decisions on the assumption that the majority of service users would require referral to secondary care, hospital-based, clinics. But if we regard psychiatric medication as a potentially useful, if sometimes problematic, element of the care plan for people struggling to cope with the stresses and pressures of normal life, it makes more sense for it to be managed by GPs as part of an overall 'psychobiosocial' care plan.

Any psychiatric medication, any professional involvement of psychiatrists (and, to be clear, all other forms of mental health care, including clinical psychologists) should be coordinated through community-based mental health and well-being teams. These teams should not only adopt a psychosocial ethos (rejecting the medical model of psychiatry), but be managed as part of local authority social services. Most of the medical aspects of this care – in relation to both mental and physical health – would best be delivered by GPs and nurses (since nursing colleagues are now competent and licensed to prescribe) attached to those community teams, rather than via the medical services of hospitals and (in the UK) NHS trusts.

A model whereby GPs provide support to community-based mental health and well-being teams would, of course, put some pressure on GPs. It would mean additional responsibilities. As we will see in a later chapter, when the economics of these plans are considered, the approach to care being discussed here would be very cost efficient. If there were a very marked reduction in the use of medication, and commensurate rationalisation of the numbers of hospital-based psychiatrists, such pressures would easily be managed. Indeed, it should be the case that increased investment in primary care would be broadly welcomed.

Appropriate models for the potential role of medical colleagues can be seen in several more visionary (and very successful) services. When describing a model service for people with very complex problems – which occasionally attract the label of 'personality disorder' – Marsha Linehan outlines the role of what she calls 'pharmacotherapists'. The service uses medical colleagues as occasional consultants to be drawn on when decisions need to be made about one small part of a wider care plan, namely the use of medication.[24] This echoes how London's Drayton Park Crisis House[25] uses its allied GP service for pragmatic prescriptions. These could, for instance, involve the short-term prescription of medication such as Zopiclone to aid sleep while a person is acutely distressed. It is important to stress that the people who use this service are experiencing serious mental health crises that would warrant hospital admission were the crisis house not available. In the UK, Tony Morrison and colleagues have recently shown that psychological therapies can be helpful for people with distressing psychotic experiences without the need to use any antipsychotic medication.[26] The Soteria project, initiated in San Jose, California, USA by the psychiatrist Loren Mosher, offers a community-based alternative to traditional psychiatry for people experiencing mental distress or in an emotional or social crisis.[27] Services based on the Soteria model and philosophy (in Sweden, Finland, Germany, Switzerland and Hungary as well as elsewhere) employ primarily non-medical staff and empha-sise the autonomy and human rights of residents. The emphasis is on preserving people's social, family and community relationships and very minimal use of antipsychotic medication. Similarly, work is also underway in the UK to find new ways to help people who have expe-rienced manic or hypomanic episodes. People are helped to identify the early warning signs of a return of a manic episode and make plans to avoid that circumstance.[28] Often, those plans involve medication (short-term medication can be effective in the early stages of a manic episode) but this is a very different prospect to the long-term, prophy-lactic, prescription of traditional psychiatry.

The next few chapters will outline what services based on these ideas might look like.

# 4
# Promote Health and Well-being

*Services should be equipped to address the full range of their clients' social, personal and psychological needs and to address both prevention and recovery. Where individual therapy is needed, effective, formulation-based, psychological therapies should be available to everyone and delivered by qualified, competent professionals. Decisions about the provision of services should be based on a person's specific problems and on the best evidence for the effectiveness of the intervention, and guided by individual formulations rather than diagnosis.*

The alternative to traditional, disease-model, mental health care that I'm outlining rejects the notion that we are (or should be) 'treating illnesses'. 'Diagnosis' is an inadequate method for describing the complex pattern of needs experienced by people in the real world, and medical accounts of 'aetiology' (medical language for causes) are misleading in attempting to explain their origins. We shouldn't make the error of assuming that our business is to 'treat illness'. Worse, with regard to social and personal problems – stressful and vulnerable employment conditions, financial austerity, social deprivation, inequalities, trauma, crime, abuse and bullying – it is wholly wrong to be aware of such threats to our well-being, but then wait until the early signs or 'symptoms' of distress to emerge before offering help. And of course it is inappropriate to have to rely on medication and other biological 'treatments'. But rather than merely complaining, we need to set out an alternative. So what *should* we do?

We should promote practical psychosocial services whose aim is to promote well-being and personal agency. That means employing community workers such as social workers, psychologists and social pedagogues (this is a role more common in Central and Northern Europe, where social pedagogues are trained in education and social psychology, and use practical educational approaches to help address a wide range of practical social welfare issues, especially for young people[1]). Such services would offer greater access to one-to-one psychotherapies of various kinds. But, vitally, they would offer primarily social solutions in the first instance. We must not make the mistake of assuming that this would mean replacing fantastic, caring, effective hospital services with trivial and ineffective social services that ignore 'real illnesses'. As we've seen, 'mental health' services simply aren't caring and effective, the disease-model approaches don't actually work very well, and social approaches are both most appropriate and most effective.

## Serious problems ... but serious social problems

Earlier, I referred to a couple of pieces of research conducted in my university department at Liverpool. To illustrate how social factors – life events and the social circumstances of our lives – can lead to personal distress, and real difficulties, I referred to Ben Barr and colleagues' research into how suicide is linked to economic recession. The links are statistically robust, and easy to understand – losing your job or feeling under the threat of redundancy can seriously affect your well-being, induce feelings of hopelessness and, clearly, lead to suicide. That is a very real and very serious outcome. Arguably, the most serious possible outcome. But this is a social phenomenon with human consequences, not a 'risk factor' for an 'illness'. I also referred to the detailed epidemiological research conducted by Richard Bentall and John Read into the impact of childhood trauma – child abuse – on the likelihood of developing psychosis. The research shows that there is a clear causal link between abuse in childhood and the experience of hallucinations or delusional beliefs in later life, and this has recently been accepted in court decisions about legal liability. These problems – often leading to the inappropriate diagnosis of 'schizophrenia' – are enormously significant for many people. That shouldn't be a surprise. Most societies take the abuse of children very seriously. Such abuse profoundly changes our relationships with parents, with other adults, our sense of self, our sense of safety and security, our understanding of the nature of adult intimate relationships. It's hardly surprising that these are considered serious crimes, and have clear links to serious psychological outcomes. But this is a social model – criminal acts impact on the victims in understandable ways.

Social issues have profound and understandable impacts on people. These are real and serious problems. But they remain social and psychological issues. This is a positive message: recognising the nature and origin of these problems allows us to see more clearly that they are understandable, preventable, amenable to change, and even more amenable if caught early.

## World Health Organization and other definitions of mental well-being

The founding Charter of the World Health Organization describes health as ' ... a state of complete physical, mental and social well-being and not merely the absence of disease or infirmity'.[2] This resonant phrase offers an indication that many medical practitioners see a focus on well-being as being central to their profession. The European Commission has gone further, and in 2001 defined mental health as ' ... a state of well-being in which the individual realizes his or her own abilities, can cope with the normal stresses of life, can work productively and fruitfully, and is able to make a contribution to his or her community.' It sees mental health as: 'a resource which enables them to realise their intellectual and emotional potential and to find and fulfil their roles in social, school and working life. For societies, good mental health of citizens contributes to prosperity, solidarity and social justice'.[3] The European Commission, interestingly, also suggests that: 'the mental condition of people is determined by a multiplicity of factors including biological (e.g., genetics, gender), individual (e.g., personal experiences), family and social (e.g., social support) and economic and environmental (e.g., social status and living conditions)'. This seems entirely compatible with the vision for psychiatry offered by Dinesh Bhugra, Pat Bracken and colleagues that I described in the introduction

I'm occasionally accused of being an incurable optimist. But it does seem to me that these approaches to the support of mental (and material) well-being are becoming key elements of government policy and professional activity. In physical health, and especially in primary care, physicians actively promote health, as well as treating illnesses. In mental health care, we see similar developments. The present UK government strategy for mental health, launched in 2011, places mental health problems in an economic context, estimating that they cost the UK at least £77 billion each year, and probably closer to £105 billion. It comments that a million people in the UK are receiving incapacity benefit, with 40% of these off work because of emotional or psychological problems, that a third of GP consultations are estimated to be as a result of mental health issues and that such problems constitute the largest proportion of 'disease burden' in public health. Finally, it discusses the physical health threats faced by people with mental health problems. This places mental health in a public health perspective, and implies a strong psychosocial ethos with an emphasis on well-being rather than 'illness'.[4]

Of course, well-being means different things to different people. The UK Office for National Statistics has the unenviable – and controversial – task of measuring well-being. The general consensus is that well-being is dependent on a broad set of issues that, taken together, determine our satisfaction with life. This offers an intriguing basis for considering what clinical psychologists or other professionals working in mental health care could consider reasonable areas for intervention.

Relationships are a vital component of well-being. That means that our social relationships with friends, our relationships with our parents, and our relationships with our children, loving or intimate relationships and relationships with work colleagues, are all important. Our physical health is important too, as is physical security – freedom from crime and the fear of crime. The quality and security of our housing is important, too – if we are homeless, live in poor-quality housing or have little security in accommodation, we're unlikely to be happy. This is equally true of our work – the extent to which our jobs are rewarding, our relationships with colleagues and bosses and the financial security that employment can bring.[5] Other aspects of well-being can include access to and appreciation of sports and leisure, and arts and culture. Most people also include our spiritual and religious lives. Perhaps two of the most important aspects of well-being are a sense of 'meaning and purpose' and active democratic political participation.

## Policies to support well-being

The main thrust of this book is to set out a new vision for mental health care whereby we move away from a 'disease-model' approach. The alternative vision that I'm offering includes a clear plan for the delivery of a range of therapeutic services. These must include one-to-one therapies, group-based therapies, novel forms of delivering therapy (for example online) and wider 'systemic' interventions such as family therapy. All these kinds of interventions aimed at helping people, families and groups to address those problems that adversely affect their mental health should be key parts of that vision. These interventions should be squarely based on a psychosocial ethos, and delivered by a broadly psychosocial multidisciplinary team. That would be a radical change. But these kinds of interventions are only part of the solution.

Decisions made by politicians and policymakers have dramatic impacts on all areas of well-being.[6] These decisions therefore have great potential for both good and ill. Obviously, political decisions can affect our wealth, and can perhaps have more impact on inequalities in wealth. That's important, because as we saw earlier, our well-being is much more closely linked to economic equality than to average economic performance.[7] Politicians in the UK also have particularly important roles in decisions about our health services: because of the unique status of our National Health Service, the decisions made by politicians have a direct effect on provision. But politicians also have a crucial role in determining our well-being through their role in changing other key social systems. Laws and related policies profoundly affect our relationships. The divorce laws, laws on same-sex marriage, pre-nuptial agreements, child-care arrangements, pension laws, benefits regulations and rules for flexible working practices all impact on relationships, and are all matters for politicians. Politicians and government departments have very significant responsibilities in shaping education and employment practice. Most education is state-funded in the UK and therefore politicians and civil servants are responsible for the range, quality and equity of education. Employment law is also very significant, and taxation rules, rules on benefits and investment decisions by government – as well as the more fundamental health of the economy – all impact on the quality of our employment and will therefore affect our well-being. Through the laws it chooses to enact, the government even affects important spiritual aspects of our lives: the role of religion in our political and cultural life, the interpretation of human rights as they apply to freedom of speech and expression. Similarly, issues related to our arts, culture and leisure are, of course, matters for government, not least through planning and investment decisions. Crime and criminal justice matters are, of course, quintessentially matters for legislators. And, finally, of course, politicians have a key role in drawing up policies and strategies in the arena of mental health. Taken together, these policies have the potential to impact profoundly on our mental health, both for good and ill.

As Pat Bracken and Dinesh Bhugra have pointed out, simplistic biomedical disease models of mental health ignore these issues. Since a person's problems are characterised as 'symptoms' of 'illness', rather than as understandable human responses to social circumstances, all these aspects of well-being, the policy decisions related to them, and the links between social circumstances and mental health are ignored or minimised. In a psychosocial model, however, these issues are integral to a full understanding of our well-being and our emotional and psychological lives.

Every responsible mental health professional believes that we should aim to prevent, rather than merely 'treat', mental health problems. This suggests that social and even political changes might be the most important targets for intervention. For example, we know that poverty is associated with mental health problems.[8] There is something grindingly awful about living each day knowing that you are unable to provide for your children's needs. All politicians aim to address poverty, but measures to reduce or eliminate poverty, especially childhood poverty, would be hugely beneficial for our mental health. However absolute income is not the only important issue. An effective way to improve our mental health would be to reduce inequality in society. We need to work together to eliminate abuses in childhood. Teachers, social workers, community nurses, GPs and the police should all try to identify and then respond to early warning signs that children might be exposed to sexual, physical or emotional abuse or neglect. Teachers and youth leaders have a role in addressing bullying in school and leisure settings. Our political leaders should also work towards less discriminatory societies, through both social and legislative actions. And, finally, many recreational drugs are associated with mental health problems. Although alcohol is unquestionably the most serious substance-related public health issue, cannabis and other recreational 'drugs' have also been associated with mental health problems. Both legal and illegal drugs are subject to laws that control their supply and use. There is clearly a role for politicians in passing legislation that could protect our health, strengthen our community, maintain our well-being and prevent mental health problems. However, in this book I'm concentrating in particular on the need for different policies regarding the delivery of mental health services, both in terms of legislation and in terms of the commissioning of services.

## Psychologists, psychiatrists, individuals and well-being

This book is intended to explain how professions such as psychiatry and clinical psychology could be reformed to reflect a psychosocial rather than a biomedical, model of mental health. I believe that both these professions are in need of reform. I discuss the implications of such a change for psychiatry throughout the book, and I devote a large part of Chapter 6 to the implications for my own profession of clinical psychology.

Clinical psychologists already offer a wide range of specialist services. They not only work in adult mental health; their skills are also important in other areas such as perinatal care, and care for expectant mothers, and in child and adolescent mental health. Psychologists work in primary care, with people with learning disabilities, and supporting patients in physical health care and physical rehabilitation services. Psychologists work with people with HIV, people with substance use problems, and in healthcare services for older adults. Many psychologists (including me) would welcome the opportunity to adopt a truly well-being focussed, psychosocial approach to our work. But this would still have significant consequences for the profession. While many of us would continue to offer one-to-one therapy, a psychosocial approach would allow for a much wider focus. That would mean working with a very wide range of community services, third sector organisations and local authority services.

I have been involved in a wide variety of different research projects over the years. One of my recent papers[9] examined how psychological processes such as rumination and self-blame are key parts of the pathway from negative life events to depression and anxiety. The two key messages from the paper are entirely consistent with the message of this book as a whole: that the events and circumstances of our lives determine our mental health (rather than some inherent personal inadequacy or genetic flaw) and that psychological processes – for example rumination – actually play a part in the chain of causes rather than merely being symptoms of 'mental disorder'.

But after that paper was published (and discussed more widely on the BBC[10]), I received a few critical questions. Although I certainly do not see things in this way, some people have commented that these kinds of psychological models could potentially be misinterpreted; seen as implying that people are in some sense responsible for their own problems because of 'errors in their thinking'. And several people asked what can be done to help?

I'm very reluctant to offer advice. It's a big subject…and if I were able to offer wise 'self-help' advice that actually worked for everybody, I'd be a millionaire. Nearly every simple piece of advice is going to be glib, obvious or wrong. But it is certainly worth thinking about how a focus on well-being could be useful. So, on my university's website, I posted some advice – advice about therapy (which I'll expand in the next chapter), and about basic support for well-being.

## Get the basics right

There are many very good reasons to look after our physical health and well-being, and maintaining our mental health is only one of them.

So it's generally a good idea to make sure that we're eating well, nutritiously, that we're keeping the saturated fat and salt content of our food low. We should – we all know – eat at least five portions of fresh fruit or vegetables a day, drink plenty of water. We should eat a balanced diet with an adequate vitamin content. We should aim to get our BMI in the healthy zone. I don't want to sound prudish, but we also know that it's good for both our mental and physical health to avoid cigarette smoke, to drink moderately and be generally quite cautious with recreational drugs. Finally, perhaps, it's valuable to make sure we get sufficient sleep – for me, at least 7 hours' sleep a night.

Although all this advice is pretty straightforward, it is all quite difficult in practice. Many people have significant problems maintaining a healthy diet and a healthy BMI. Many people smoke, drink to excess and many people take recreational drugs of many different kinds. This is where the links between mental and physical health become important. This is also where the services offered by GP colleagues come into their own, and where the benefits of a community-based service are perhaps most obvious. It is very difficult for people to make all these changes in their lives, and yet they can be profoundly important in promoting and protecting their mental and physical health.

There is a great deal of advice and specific help that health services can offer here. These can be augmented by, and are often integrated with, the services of local authorities, charities and third-sector organisations. Depending on our individual circumstances, we can access a range of services to address diet, over-eating (and other food-related difficulties) and exercise. We have access to services to help people quit smoking, address alcohol problems, and come off street drugs and prescription medication. We have exercise classes of many kinds. We have breast-feeding support groups, and sleep clinics. Occasionally these are provided by government organisations such as the NHS, sometimes they are provided by third-sector organisations or by the local authorities. I can entirely understand frustration from people who have found it difficult to access these services – we need significant investment in these kinds of basic, preventative, services. I believe that successful investment in these kinds of basic physical well-being services could very substantially reduce the burden on secondary care services in both physical and mental health. But whether we're arguing that people should avail themselves of the services that are on offer, or arguing that there should be much greater investment in these services, the message is the same…get the basic, physical, fundamentals right.[11]

## Five ways to mental well-being

Moving from physical health to mental well-being, there are plenty of straightforward things people can do. A recent UK Government report into well-being commissioned a team at the new economics foundation to find evidence for things individuals could do themselves to achieve greater well-being. They concluded that we would be well-advised to follow a well-being equivalent of the 'five fruit and vegetables a day' rule.[12]

### 1.   Be active...

The links between physical activity and increased well-being are clear, so taking part in physical exercise on a regular basis obviously makes sense. Activity improves our mood as well as making us healthier and increasing our psychological well-being. It changes our brain chemistry, boosting levels of the neurotransmitters that make us feel good. Exercise, in fact, is a good example of how biological factors can influence our psychological processes. However, it is also important to remember that people differ in their levels of physical fitness and health. Any advice on keeping active and fit has to be tailored to each individual. It is a good idea to take advice from professionals such as a fitness coach, a physiotherapist or your GP. But all of us can take steps to ensure we keep physically fit and active every day: going for a walk, or perhaps taking the dog out for a walk (if you don't have a dog, get one!). If the opportunity is there, go to the gym. Try going for a run, a swim or a cycle ride. Even just doing the gardening or DIY is great, it ensures you stay active and will raise your mood as well as keep you fit. Dancing is very good... although personally I have to confess that I am far too self-conscious even to contemplate dancing. Regardless of what exercise you choose, the point is that activity makes you feel good.

Activity also helps with our sleep. Sleep problems are very common, and can have a significant impact on well-being. People who are sleep deprived often feel miserable, irritable and, of course, tired and lethargic. Evidence suggests that sleep is important for your physical health – especially your immune system. Sleep is important, and exercise is a good way to help ensure that you sleep well. As I will explain in a moment, our relationships are important for our well-being, and many forms of physical activity are communal – people join sports clubs or teams. For example, my son is engaged in football teams and cycling clubs. So a commitment to physical activity can have knock-on benefits.

## 2. Connect...

Our relationships are fundamentally important to our well-being. Although it is difficult to compare the relative importance of different elements of well-being, we are quintessentially social animals, and it is not unreasonable to claim that relationships may well be the most important overall contributors to happiness. Loving partnerships, sexual relationships, but also parental relationships, relationships with friends, with work colleagues and with neighbours are all important. Because of the close link between relationships and well-being, it's worth investing time and effort to maintain our connections with the people around us. Good, supportive relationships (which will mean different things to different people) are contributors to happier, healthier and longer lives. In fact, loneliness may pose a risk to our health similar to that of smoking and over-eating, two huge health concerns. Relationships and the social support that they can bring appear to protect us from infection, lower our risk of heart disease and reduce the chances of developing dementia in old age. For me as a psychologist, it's clear that our self esteem and our sense of self-worth develop in relationships – through how other people view us, how they feel about us. It is also important that people have a sense of belonging; to feel that they fit into a community. And there are things that we can do to support this. Simple practical steps towards greater connectivity can be made by anyone. We can do new things such as join groups and organisations, but we can also make sure we maintain the relationships we already have – keeping in contact with the people close to us.

## 3. Keep learning...

Keeping mentally active keeps you happy. Continuing with learning and staying curious and engaged may make us better equipped to deal with life's challenges. Learning new skills also gives people a sense of achievement, which in turn can boost our self-confidence and self-esteem. Again, there are many practical things we can do to keep mentally active. As an academic, I tend to recommend things like the Open University. But formal qualifications are not the only available options. The 'five ways to well-being' suggest we should: '...try something new. Rediscover an old interest. Sign up for that course. Take on a different responsibility at work. Fix a bike. Learn to play an instrument or how to cook your favourite food. Set a challenge you enjoy achieving...' All of which I believe is excellent advice.

This is the perfect opportunity to mention The Reader Organisation.[13] The Reader Organisation is a social enterprise dedicated to literature.

Its members organise reading groups within the health service, the criminal justice system, emergency services, work places, care homes, looked-after children's services and many more. These reading groups are primarily opportunities for people to experience reading together, as a group. People are encouraged to read aloud and discuss together the ways that great literature can affect their mood and perspectives on life. These reading groups, and related activities such as community theatre projects, have been a huge success and are greatly appreciated by participants; perhaps this is because the community-based activities run by the Reader organisation seem to address many of the steps to well-being which are the focus of this chapter.

### 4.   Give ...

Human beings have evolved as part of communities: and being part of good, supportive relationships are key to our survival. Good supportive relationships are reciprocal and whilst receiving support and care makes us feel good, so does caring for others. As Action for Happiness puts it: '...caring about others is fundamental to our happiness...'. Doing things for other people is a very powerful way to feel happier and can improve mental well-being.

There are many ways of giving. Many of us give money to charity, but the giving I'm talking about here is wider than this. We can give our time, ideas, energy, enthusiasm and leadership. This doesn't have to be a big thing, or even a regular commitment. We can ensure – in the spirit of 'five a day' – that we do at least something every day to boost well-being: small, often unplanned acts to help strangers, family, friends, colleagues or neighbours. Even a small gesture such as giving someone directions to their destination can make us feel good. These suggestions are not merely nice ideas. Research evidence shows that helping others improves our own happiness. Helping other people can lead to supportive reciprocal relationships, increase our own feelings of competence, improve our mood and reduce stress.

### 5.   Take notice ...

The fifth 'step to happiness' may not be as obvious to everyone as the previous four. Mindfulness is defined as 'the state of being attentive to, and aware of, what is taking place in the present'. To be mindful is to be consciously and intentionally aware of what is happening around us as well as what is going on in our minds (our thoughts and feelings). The ability to be mindful can be learned, and has been shown to have significant benefits for our mental well-being and physical health. Mindfulness is particularly effective in dealing with stress; it helps people relax and can improve sleep. Not only does mindfulness reduce feelings of stress, it can also improve our relationships by increasing our levels of empathy and compassion.

The idea of 'mindfulness' can be a difficult, abstract idea for people to grasp. To cultivate a mindful stance, we do not necessarily need to go on a training course on mindfulness, although that wouldn't be a bad idea. However, we can also take easy steps in everyday life to encourage an open-minded, curious mental approach.[14] The new economics foundation advises us to: 'catch sight of the beautiful. Remark on the unusual. Notice the changing seasons. Savour the moment, whether you are walking to work, eating lunch or talking to friends. Be aware of the world around you and what you are feeling. Reflecting on your experiences will help you appreciate what matters to you.' One common tip to increase mindfulness is to focus briefly on your breathing; to stop what you're doing and to concentrate on all the feelings and sensations involved – the feeling of your chest inflating, the cool air entering your nose, the pressure as you hold your breath and the warm air on your top lip as you breath out. The point is that the brief pause, and the focussed concentration is a calming, mindful experience. A slightly different, but also mindful, experience might be the morning coffee taken in the garden watching the birds busying themselves and feeling the sun on your face (often something we recognise from holidays or Sunday mornings).

## Psychological processes

I realise that we sometimes tend to blame others for the way they think about themselves, other people, the world and the future. The insulting label of 'personality disorder', for example, paradoxically manages to both label people as 'ill' and at the same time blame them for their ways of thinking. As a cognitive psychologist, I recognise that how we make sense of the world is important. But I also know that we LEARN to make sense of the world. All the things that have happened to me in my life – my biological inheritance, my parenting, the social circumstances and cultural values around me as I grew up, my education and, vitally, the life events and traumas that I have lived through – have all shaped my views on life. My view of the world, and the ways I tend to think (including my tendency to ruminate) are obviously shaped by the journey I've taken through life. So I do think that the ways that people think about the world is important – the evidence points that out very clearly – but there are perfectly understandable reasons why people have learned to look at the world in the ways they do.

But also...what can be done about it? What can we do to change our ways of thinking? One of the important implications of the research I mentioned earlier is that if we were able to 'turn off' the rumination and self-blame, we'd be able to 'turn down' at least some of the depression and anxiety. That's really the basis of clinical psychology – while there are very good reasons why we each learn our own particular way of making sense of things, sometimes it might be a good idea to see if we can develop new ways to engage with the world, especially in stressful times.

## Psychological therapy is not a different kind of drug

We have known for thousands of years that talking through our understanding of a situation can be helpful. The ancient Greeks believed that philosophers could offer very real comfort to people in distress, and I myself found what amounts to a fictionalised account of cognitive behavioural therapy in an obscure old English poem – '*The Regement of Princes*' – from the year 1411.[15] But it is over the past few decades – really since the Second World War – that we've seen the most major proliferation of psychological therapies. I am strongly of the opinion that this is a very good thing, but also that we need to think in a cool-headed fashion about the fundamental nature and substance of psychological therapy.

I believe it bears repetition to say that our emotions and behaviour (and therefore our mental health) are largely determined by how we make sense of and understand the world. That is, in turn, largely determined by our experiences and upbringing. Biological, social and circumstantial factors affect our mental health partly through their effect on psychological processes. And therefore, at least for me, it makes sense to try to understand how our psychology 'works'. Although I am no great fan of the idea that people's problems are the result of 'thinking errors', I do think it makes sense in some situations to see if we can help people understand their world and the things that have happened to them in different ways. When people are lonely and frightened, they may come to believe the situation is hopeless. Children exposed to abuse often come to believe that they are responsible in some way for the things that have happened to them. In short, there are whole swathes of ways in which people – all of us – think irrationally. Occasionally, those understandable irrationalities can lead to, or keep us stuck in, significant emotional distress. It seems entirely reasonable that discussing with caring, knowledgeable therapists the ways in which we make sense of the world can sometimes help us look at the world differently...and this can sometimes be helpful.

There is, of course, widespread debate over the effectiveness of psychological therapies in general, and researchers actively debate the relative effectiveness of different styles of therapy. I am a practising clinical psychologist, and occasionally I use schema-focussed cognitive behavioural therapy. In part, my professional orientation is based on my reading of the available literature. The wide range of problems subsumed under the general topic of 'mental health' means nobody can claim to have fingertip access to all the relevant research. We are aware of the emerging trends, and most importantly, we know where to go to obtain the most up-to-date information.

In the UK, as we discussed briefly in the previous chapter, the National Institute for Health and Care Excellence or NICE[16] is charged with offering independent, authoritative and evidence-based guidance on the most effective ways to prevent, diagnose and treat disease and ill-health, promote well-being and reduce inequalities in healthcare and health outcomes. Its principal mechanism for this is the publication of clinical guidelines. These guidelines give advice to clinicians about the best way to manage health conditions, and advise commissioners as to which approaches are most cost-effective. They therefore, of course, also offer members of the public access to high-quality information on which to base decisions about their own health. The guidelines are developed through a process of systematic review of the available published literature, especially clinical trials, and represent something of an expert consensus as to the effectiveness of different interventions.

For all the difficulties regarded as mental health problems, psychological interventions of one kind or another are recommended to clinicians and commissioners. This means that the professional and scientific consensus, based upon systematic review of the published results of randomised controlled trials, is that such psychological therapies are not only effective, but also cost-effective. That's good news for psychologists (it would be a little challenging, emotionally, if any of our interventions, including therapy, were deemed to be ineffective). And it is broadly good news that we are seeing increasing investment in such services. But this approach, predicated on the disease model of psychiatry, nevertheless has its problems and in my opinion needs further reform.

## IAPT – Improving Access to Psychological Therapies

On 12 May 2006, the UK Secretary of State for Health, Patricia Hewitt and her Care Services Minister, Rosie Winterton, issued a press release entitled 'End of the "prozac nation" – More counselling, more therapy, less medication to treat depression'.[17] This announced a very ambitious plan substantially to increase the funding of psychological therapies in the UK. In the UK, of course, such services are provided free at the point of need, and therefore need to be commissioned. The government programme launched in 2006 eventually saw nearly £1 billion invested in psychological therapies. In order to ensure that this money was spent on such therapies and not absorbed without visible effect in the general running costs of the National Health Service, there was a separate procurement and commissioning process. It was called the Improving Access to Psychological Therapies Programme, or IAPT. Guided by the evidence supplied by NICE, the National Institute for Health and Care Excellence, the programme aimed to focus in its initial phase on the provision of one particular type of psychological therapy for one group of clients – cognitive behavioural therapy (or CBT) for adults of working age experiencing mild to moderate anxiety or depression.

An important theme in the IAPT programme is the way in which services are commissioned. In order to ensure that the programme delivered what was intended, people were invited to tender for very specific service contracts. These covered both the delivery of the psychotherapy services and the training of the therapists. The declared aim of the programme[18] was to train an extra 10,000 'therapists'. These were intended to be a mix of clinical psychologists (the early plans, soon dropped, were to see a large increase in the number of clinical psychologists in the NHS) and specialist CBT therapists. A bespoke training scheme was begun, with very detailed specifications for the competencies that were needed.

The IAPT programme has been controversial. Initial reports of success have been followed with accounts of satisfactory, but not outstanding, performance. The numbers involved are impressive, with many hundreds of thousands of people receiving CBT. Many people – including many clinical psychologists – have praised the programme. But there have been criticisms, too. The overtly political nature of the programme has been controversial. Many psychologists and therapists regard themselves as advocates of their clients, and some were unhappy that the overt aims of the IAPT programme included a return to work and consequent reduction in benefits costs. CBT itself is somewhat controversial. Many critics point again to the political background to the IAPT programme, and suggest that people's emotional distress, and indeed any thinking styles that accompany this distress, originate in the social, financial and economic circumstances of people's lives. In that context, many people suggest that to focus on what goes on inside people's heads, rather than addressing the causes of their distress, risks missing the point. Some even see it as blaming the victims. Many critics of the IAPT programme argue that government action should have been predicated not on attempting to treat so-called 'mental disorders' in people who have been rendered desperate by economic circumstances, but instead on helping people challenge and respond to those economic and social circumstances directly. In this context, many people find CBT to be a 'sticking-plaster' solution.

## Thinking errors?

Of course, supporters of CBT argue differently. They suggest that CBT directly addresses key psychological, rather than political or social, problems. In a multi-disciplinary team, they argue, social and financial problems can, or at least should be, dealt with – and dealt with by professionals other than clinical psychologists with the appropriate skills for the task. Many would argue that, whilst political and social change is needed, our individual professional responsibilities are somewhat different. We may, to use an analogy, lobby politicians for changes to road traffic regulations, but that shouldn't prevent paramedics offering medical help at a road traffic collision. Although 'CBT' is a very broad term, the theoretical assumptions underlying at least some versions of the therapeutic approach are seen by some as problematic. Typically, CBT therapists help their clients become aware of the links between their thinking styles and their emotions. So, for example, someone may say that they feel depressed after receiving a piece of equivocal feedback, and also that '...nothing I ever do is good enough'. Therapy continues, predictably, with the therapist helping the client realise the links between this style of thinking and the consequent emotions, and to identify other possible ways of seeing the situation. And therein lies a further potential source of controversy. Although not all would agree, many psychologists and psychotherapists worry that CBT can give people the message that they are to blame for their difficulties because they are in some sense 'thinking wrong' or making 'thinking errors' which need to be corrected through therapy. This is contentious.

## A new approach to psychological therapies

Psychological therapy is a not a like-for-like replacement for medication. Part of the problems with the IAPT programme and with the widespread growth in the use of CBT is that we often talk as if 'CBT for depression' is conceptually the same as 'antidepressants for depression'. Unfortunately, too many psychologists are complicit with this idea. Our psychological well-being – our mental health – is dependent (at least in large part) on our framework of understanding about ourselves, other people, the world and the future. This framework of understanding does not represent some form of 'pathology' or 'thinking error', but rather the natural and understandable consequence of events and experiences in our lives together with our learned responses to those events. In that context, helping people to learn more resilient ways of responding to the challenges of the work can be useful. We need to talk to people and to try to understand their perspectives, the way they see the world, the messages that they have taken away from things that have happened to them, and how they approach the challenges in their lives. We need to work collaboratively with people to develop new ways of responding, and to examine the evidence for the conclusions they have drawn. When someone loses their job and concludes that there is no point in living, we should explore with them why they might have reached that conclusion ... and help them get a job. When an abused child comes to believe that she is responsible for the abuse, that she is unlovable and evil, we should challenge that conclusion ... but at the same time actively help protect children from abuse and bring abusers to justice. But we should not be under the misapprehension that these conversations, however helpful they might be, represent a set of 'treatments' for 'pathologies'. There is no such thing as 'abnormal psychology' just as there is no such thing as 'abnormal physics'.

And that means that all psychological therapies should all be based on intelligent integration of evidence about which approaches seem to be most helpful in general, and about how they impact on psychological processes (such as the tendency to interpret things in certain ways). Of course, all psychological therapies should be delivered by qualified, competent professionals. Decisions about what therapy or therapies should be offered to whom should be based their specific problems and on the best evidence is about what is likely to help with those problems, not on diagnosis. Individual formulations should be used to put together an individualised package of care suitable for addressing each person's unique set of problems. Since even clinical psychologists currently often follow a tacit disease model, using psychological therapies as part of a psychosocial, rather than biomedical, ethos would significantly change the way that clinical psychologists and others work.

With a starting point of a simple list of problems (as discussed in Chapter 2), the clinician and client should work together to come up with a shared understanding of the nature, causes and possible solutions for those problems – an individual case formulation. Each profession uses the term 'formulation', but each a little differently. It is common for psychiatrists, for example, to refer to a formulation developed *after* a diagnosis has been given – in other words, the client's problems will be assessed, the most appropriate diagnostic label agreed upon and then a more fulsome account of social and psychological aspects will be developed. Clearly, in the approach recommended here, such formulations should predominantly focus on the social and psychological contributors to a person's distress. Clinical psychologists, on the other hand, see formulations as alternatives to (rather than additions to) diagnosis. The formulations of clinical psychologists – with which I am, naturally, most familiar – usually consist of a list of problems together with hypotheses as to the possible origins of those problems. Good formulations should be based on a coherent 'psychobiosocial' model. That is, they should attempt to identify which of the almost infinite set of possible social, environmental and biological factors might be playing a role. We should attempt to identify factors in a person's childhood: parental absence or bereavement; emotional, physical or sexual abuse; bullying or abuse in childhood; the attachment relationships with parents; key life events... the list is a long one. We should also attempt to identify those social factors known to lead to mental health problems in adulthood: marital difficulties, loneliness, unemployment and its mirror – unrewarding, insecure, stressful or bullying jobs – and financial difficulties. Again, the list is a long one. We should equally attempt to identify those very many biological factors that could influence a person's mental health – whether they be familial traits (of which I, personally, am highly sceptical, as they seem most highly likely to be family myths rather than real biological vulnerabilities and which may, in any case, represent learned patterns rather than biological pathologies) or physical ailments that understandably affect our psychological well-being. This is not intended to be a guide for conducting psychological therapy. This is not an extensive list of all the areas that need to be considered when assessing possible causal factors. It is merely intended to give an idea of those challenging events and circumstances that can lead to mental health problems and should be part of any assessment process.

Psychological accounts of mental health problems do not see people as mere corks, bobbed around by the waves of circumstance, neither do they see people as the product of biology alone. Instead, people make sense of their world, actively interpreting events and then responding to them. As well as assessing biological ('nature') and environmental ('nurture') factors in the development of mental health problems, psychologists quintessentially must explore the person's individual psychological response to events.[19]

It is an unfortunate concomitant of the growth in CBT over the past few years that appreciation of, and emphasis on our shared and normal psychological mechanisms seems to have shrunk rather than grown. This could be a consequence of the fact that, encouraged by the IAPT programme, many of the CBT therapists now practicing in the UK and abroad do not have a first degree in psychology. This makes their practice somewhat manual-based and naturally renders them less able to identify (or even recognise) key psychological mechanisms and their importance. In many descriptions of CBT for the public, emphasis is placed on the links between our thoughts and our mood, and reference is often made to 'negative automatic thoughts'. Psychological science is much richer than this. Again, an exhaustive list of psychological mechanisms and the ways in which quirks in the details of these mechanisms can affect our understanding of the world and interpretation of events would be much too long for this book. But psychologists can draw on knowledge of our perceptual system and the way that we make sense of the huge volume of visual and auditory information hitting our eyes and ears every second. We understand how people make sense of this information and how the brain stores information in memory. We understand basic principles of reward and punishment, and the details of how such technical issues as 'discriminant stimuli' and 'intermittent reinforcement' can make certain behaviours extremely difficult to change. Complex theoretical models such as the 'interacting cognitive subsystems' model[20] can help to understand how the human mind transforms structural information about the world (the patterns of light and dark, edges and corners) into, first, factual information, then, progressively, information concerning objects, people, actions, relationships, and finally intentions and meaning, including emotional meaning. This touches on the striking phenomenon of 'change blindness', where people simply fail to notice significant changes in the real world.[21] We have detailed (and constantly evolving) theoretical insights into the ways in which people understand their relationships with parents, with peers, partners and others. We study how people understand and explain events in the outside world: the 'causal attributions' we make about events seem to be particularly important not only for guiding our actions but also for our mental well-being – and how we identify and appraise our own internal physical states. There is a large and growing literature on how we understand our own thoughts – an area of research obviously closely linked to the idea of 'mindfulness'. Psychologists have studied a wide range of mental processes related to how we form and maintain beliefs, which is obviously pertinent to a wide range of serious mental health problems. Psychologists have studied – have won Nobel prizes for studying – 'heuristic reasoning', that is the mental 'short-cuts' that we use to make sense of and act towards a complex universe where much is possible and little is certain.[22] We know a great deal about how people develop their sense of self, and how they maintain their self-esteem when things go wrong. Psychologists, especially from behavioural tradition, understand how people and animals respond in circumstances of unremitting punishment (so-called 'learned helplessness'). More recent 'cognitive' research (that is, research studying thinking processes) has explored our sense of self-efficacy (what we believe we can do, and why) and the negative cognitive schemas (sets of related thoughts) that accompany the depressed mood.

In a genuinely psychological approach, therapy should then proceed on the basis of these identified psychological processes (and this is, again, a very sketchy and inadequate illustrative list). In a genuinely 'psychobiosocial' model, we would see a genuine assessment of possible biological factors that could be playing a role, and the consideration of the possible role of medication. More pertinently in most cases, we would see a comprehensive assessment of the person's social circumstances and a practical, integrated, plan to address these real-world issues. For me, as a psychologist, we would also see a research-informed analysis of the possible role played by the way that the person is making sense of their world, and whether they are interested in exploring possibilities for change in that respect.

In practice, this rarely happens, even in the CBT of the IAPT programme. Despite the dominant role of psychiatry in the current mental health system, the basics of biomedicine are often neglected. People in the mental health system often have very poor physical health, sometimes exacerbated by poverty, loneliness, hopelessness, and the physically damaging effects of the medication. Those are surely matters for our medical colleagues. In passing, I believe that the failure of biomedical psychiatry to address these health issues is another very good reason to envision a much greater role for GPs. More specifically to mental health, it is currently the case that the very biomedical aspects of a case formulation that are argued to give our medical colleagues 'clinical primacy' in the care team are often neglected. Quite aside from the shameful failure to give all clients proper medical care, the biomedical aspects of clients' mental health issues are usually explored in a very cursory fashion. There is a good reason for this – MRI scans or blood tests are pretty much worthless in psychiatry; we (unsurprisingly, given my arguments so far) simply do not have biomarkers for mental health problems. As a consequence, in practice the role of the biomedical specialist defaults to making inaccurate, unreliable and invalid diagnoses and issuing prescriptions for psychiatric drugs which, as we saw in the previous chapter, bear little systematic relationship to the diagnosis, are in no real sense 'cures' and seem to cause nearly as many problems as they solve, at least in the long run.

Services commissioned through the IAPT programme may not meet the needs of our GP colleagues in their primary medical role either. Although I am no supporter of biomedical dominance, initiatives such as IAPT – indeed many initiatives involving secondary-care services to which GPs refer, rather than services within primary care – may make this neglect of physical health and genuine psychiatry even worse. Instead of community mental health and well-being teams with close links to primary care, as I would advocate, access to CBT and other psychological therapies too often relies on referral. The client is referred to an external service. While the GP (or another referrer) has determined that the person requires psychological therapy, the practical consequence is a referral to a service outside of the primary care system, in which – typically – a therapist engages in conventional CBT as a stand-alone intervention. Even if that therapist were medically trained (an extreme rarity), the nature of the service and the intent of the referral preclude any assessment of physical health. In practice, then, services such as the CBT provision commissioned under the IAPT programme often fail to consider physical health needs or any biological factors which may be playing a role in someone's mental health problems. Our system urgently needs reform.

The same considerations apply to the second major set of causal agents – social factors. In an ideal system, a comprehensive assessment of the client's social needs would contribute to the care plan, and assertive action would ensue. Theoretically, the major causal factors involved in someone's mental health problems should be identified, and careful, detailed and expert care taken to identify the pathways from external crisis – abuse, poverty, loneliness, unemployment, debt and so on – to understandable emotional distress. Practically, solutions should be developed that address these root causes. But instead of this, the referral to separate, secondary-care services such as those commissioned under the IAPT scheme can all too often effectively ignore such social factors. Public statements will refer to the ways in which local authority social services departments should work with mental health services to provide integrated care. In practice, these issues are quietly sidelined. The dominant biomedical model minimises (often, tacitly, by neglect) the role of social factors. CBT therapists are usually untrained in such social factors.

Instead of addressing the three aspects of a biopsychosocial or a psychobiosocial model in an integrated way, all too often 'psychological therapy' services provided through programmes such as IAPT merely offer clients a standardised, one-size-fits-all, manual-based, surface-level, sticking-plaster pseudo-solution. The therapists are trained and competent in delivering standard CBT. And that has its merits. But they are usually untrained in assessing and addressing biological, factors as part of a comprehensive formulation of a person's needs. They are usually equally untrained in assessing and addressing social factors. Perhaps most depressingly, they are often largely untrained in the final – psychological – element. There is a difference between understanding the complex psychological processes that pertain to an individual's circumstances and applying one of a limited number of standard CBT protocols (one for 'depression', one for 'generalised anxiety', one for 'panic disorder' and so on).

## Two steps forwards, only one step back

The ideal model for mental health services would be for community mental health and well-being services, based on a psychosocial ethos and managed within local authority social services, to be integrated with primary care GP services. In such a system, GPs would assess the biological aspects of problems and whether, and which, medication might be helpful. We would offer a comprehensive assessment of people's social circumstances and a practical, integrated, plan to address these real-world issues. We would offer a research-informed analysis of the possible role played by the way that the person is making sense of their world, and potential avenues for change in this respect. Where does the CBT offered by programmes such as IAPT fit in that picture?

We are clearly not there yet. Further radical reform is needed. CBT as experienced by too many people at present is nowhere near that ideal. Because it is offered within a health service dominated by a medical ethos, and wedded to diagnosis, people access services not on the basis of need, but on the basis of diagnosis. Services are informed by clinical guidelines that, themselves, tend to rely on diagnosis. Despite the media release accompanying the initial launch of the IAPT programme, the number of prescriptions for antidepressants is rising, not falling. And when referred for psychological interventions, people are still receiving a standardised 'package' of therapy that resembles a non-medical anti-depressant. There is, incidentally, considerable evidence that CBT thera-pists within the IAPT programme find it very difficult to stick to their brief. Web-based forums on which CBT therapists discuss their experi-ences reveal that the people who actually use IAPT are often not those envisaged in the plan. Although the service remains focussed on adults of working age, it is clear that the range of problems that people bring is very broad, including long-standing relationship difficulties, prob-lems with substance use and serious mental health problems. In conse-quence, straightforward CBT is often inappropriate ... and therapists are often frustrated by the narrowness of their training.

Significant investment in effective psychological therapies should be seen as a good thing, and the IAPT programme should be welcomed. If it is imperfect, it should be regarded as a stepping-stone to something better. I cautiously welcome current government plans in the UK for the future of psychological therapies.[23] Although it is sad to see that additional, ring-fenced, funding for psychological therapies is to be substantially reduced, there seems to be a high level of commitment to commission psychological therapies, and the essential nature of psycho-logical therapy services seems to be evolving in a positive direction.

## Psychological therapies as part of integrated services

Expansion of the provision of psychological therapies such as CBT has the potential to liberate many thousands of people from misery. But we should not think of emotional distress as a symptom of 'illness' and 'prescribe' CBT as if it were some form of drug. Since the ways in which people make sense of the world and respond to challenging circum-stances are primary determinants of their mental health and well-being, these are reasonable targets for a therapeutic response. It can clearly prove useful to help people identify the lens through which they see the world – how they think about themselves, other people, the world and the future – how and why they have developed that particular perspec-tive, and what impact that has. It is equally useful to explore the prac-tical applications of this approach, helping people to learn new ways of looking at the world. But there's much more to a psychological approach than 'talking treatments' for 'mental disorder'.

We need significant investment in psychological approaches, including CBT. But this is not enough. Services should be designed such that all aspects of a person's mental health needs can be assessed and addressed. This would include comprehensive assessment of physical health and consideration of the possible role of medication. This should be integrated with an equally comprehensive assessment of the person's social circumstances and a practical, integrated, plan to address these real-world issues. Of course, as a psychologist, I am bound to argue that we also need to understand how the person is making sense of their world and consider what could be done to help them change either their understanding of the world or to develop more appropriate responses. But I am also saying that we need to start thinking a little differently about CBT itself. CBT is effective because it is a systematic way of helping us reflect on our own thought processes and, if necessary, changing them. This is not merely a form of 'talking treatment'. It is the practical application of the fact that our mental health is largely dependent on our understanding of the world, our thoughts about ourselves, other people, the future, and the world.

# 5
# Residential Care ... Not Medical Coercion

*When people are in crisis, they may need residential care, but this should not be seen as a medical issue. Hospitals should therefore be replaced with residential units designed and managed from a psychosocial perspective. Medical expertise may well be an important part of the service, but medical colleagues should act as consultants to the team, not be seen having sapiential authority over the team. In cases where, regrettably, the powers of the Mental Health Act are needed and compulsion is required, any decisions we take should be subject to judicial oversight and based on the risks that individuals pose to themselves and others, together with their capacity to make decisions about their own care, rather than whether or not they are considered 'mentally ill'.*

I have spent my career divided between clinical and academic work. Much of my work has been focussed on in-patient settings and with people who have quite severe and disabling problems. After qualifying, I divided my working week between in-patient, hospital-based, psychiatric ward and an out-patient clinic. When I conducted my PhD, I spent a great deal of my time interviewing people who were resident on in-patient psychiatric wards. In my academic career, I have been responsible for randomised, controlled trials of CBT for people with serious mental health problems: this again frequently brought me into contact with people staying in hospital. And throughout my career I have continued to work with people with serious problems, who are often frequently admitted to hospital. But I have to confess that I had not visited a psychiatric ward for several months until recently, when one of my clients was briefly admitted to hospital. And I was, again, shocked by her experience.

The details of my client's mental health problems are not relevant here, but, like many people who are admitted to psychiatric hospitals, she had been experiencing problems for a number of years. From time to time, the challenges of caring for her became too much for her parents, and (occasionally following the intervention of the police) she spent a few days in hospital. It is significant for the narrative of this book that there has never been a dramatic change in the care offered during her admissions – no new diagnosis, no new or insightful formulation, no change in prescription – the main reason for her admission is to provide some respite for her parents. So this particular admission was not unusual. In truth, my client welcomed it. Her anxieties were such that admission to hospital represented 'safety' for her. The point of this story is to capture my impression on visiting her. My first impression wasn't great. I had expected to walk in, to be greeted by a nurse or other healthcare worker and, within the sensible parameters of visiting regulations, spend time with the person I had come to visit. I had expected the environment to be inappropriately medical, but I expected clinical cleanliness and tidiness. Instead, I was confronted by a peculiar 'air-lock' style arrangement – I entered through a conventional automatic, sliding, door, but had to wait until that door had closed, and locked, behind me. Then a security guard – not a receptionist – asked me my business. I said I was a friend of a patient (the guard asked for her name) and was asked to give my name before being issued with a visitor's badge and the second automatic door was opened. I was already uncomfortable – my client was a voluntary patient, she had not been detained under the Mental Health Act and was therefore – in theory at least – entirely free to come and go as she wished. In my opinion, that right should extend to her visitors. I can, of course, see why psychiatric units need to consider security, but the immediate impression was unpleasant. The theme was immediately one of risk, dangerousness, threat. Certainly not one of calm. I made my way to the ward, and, once through the main doors, there was no immediate sense of control or coercion. I met my client in a general activity room, but there was an odd, institutional feel. The unit was busy, even crowded. There were some comfortable chairs, but they were upholstered in a plasticised material – the kind you find on the chairs in an Accident and Emergency waiting area. In any case, the only space that my client and I could find was sitting in upright chairs at a table – which obviously doubled as a dining unit. There were artworks on the walls, but there were also boards for posters, information leaflets and health-related messages. Those of us who work in, or visit, psychiatric wards will recognise this picture. I have a different vision.

## A place of safety

In England and Wales, care for people with mental health problems is overseen (in large part) by the Mental Health Act (2007).[1] The Act refers to a 'place of safety' – a legal term that has been in use in the UK for many years. Two sections of the Act give police officers power to move a person whom they believe to have a mental health problem to a 'place of safety'. Interestingly (in the light of arguments I shall make below), if the person in question is not in a 'public place', the police officers must obtain a warrant (issued by a magistrate – a UK term referring to a form of junior judge) before taking this course of action. Detailed advice to police officers, issued by the UK Home Office, makes it clear that 'places of safety' would normally be considered to be hospitals, other medical facilities, residential care homes or the home of a relative or friend. It is common, however for people who are thought to be under the influence of alcohol or recreational drugs, rather than suffering from a mental health problem, to be taken into police custody.

So, then, if we were in crisis, what would we consider to be a 'place of safety'? What would we want in such circumstances? Perhaps, let's be clear about what isn't needed. People in acute distress are not 'ill' and do not need to be in 'hospital'. I am aware that this is a challenging thing to say. But I mean precisely what I say. As I made clear in Chapters 2 and 3, 'illness' and 'diagnosis' are inappropriate metaphors for understanding emotional distress. When problems are serious or acute, people can certainly need help, and occasionally medication can be useful. But they aren't 'ill' and there is no good reason to suppose that a 'hospital' is the most appropriate place of safety. Instead, people deserve to be offered a high quality, welcoming, supportive and calm environment in which to recover and receive the help they need.

## Physical health

Many colleagues' immediate concerns on hearing the suggestion that we drop the notion of hospital admission for people who need residential care – whether on a short-term or long-term basis – will be anxiety about a person's physical health.

It is absolutely true that people with mental health problems often have major physical health problems too. It is certainly true that admission to a psychiatric hospital offers, in theory, an opportunity to help clients access the help – the physical healthcare – that they need. But, in practice, people at present find it difficult to access such help, despite being an in- or out-patient in a 'hospital'. The conclusion has to be that hospital care is failing even in that respect.

To put some flesh on those bones of an argument: in the UK, both the Royal College of Psychiatrists and the Department of Health have expressed serious concerns over the physical health of, and physical healthcare provided to, people in residential psychiatric care. There are two obvious issues here – the identification of relevant medical conditions at admission, especially medical conditions that might help explain a person's problems, and on-going physical health care of residents. It is important to understand and then address any medical conditions that might affect our mental health. In truth, however, these are rare. Despite the frantic assertions of the pharmaceutical companies, the emotional and social problems labelled as 'mental health problems' are primarily just that – social and psychological issues. Although we cannot – and should not try to – separate our physical from our mental health, that is simply not the same as assuming that mental health problems are 'illnesses' and that they should be treated as such. So it is very rare indeed for physical health problems to be the primary causes of mental health problems.

People do not reach the doors of psychiatric wards without first having contact with a number of health and social care staff. The majority of people admitted to hospital are already known to the services, whose needs and care plans are understood, but whose social circumstances are such that, at least occasionally, they need additional support. Many people are in acute crises, and access services through Accident and Emergency departments, following calls to the ambulance services or via the police. In such circumstances, it is indeed important that people have their primary medical needs assessed. About ten years ago, I worked as a clinical psychologist on a 'psychiatric intensive care unit'. One Monday morning, we held our usual 'ward round' (and, yes, of course we definitely need to change that terminology) and were updated on a young man who had been admitted over the weekend. The psychiatric registrar reported (rather proudly) that the young man had been brought into the unit late on the Friday afternoon by an ambulance crew after his friends had reported that he had been acting very oddly in a Gestalt therapy session – he began speaking incoherently and defecated in public. Understandably, his behaviour led to an immediate emergency call and – because he was extremely uncooperative with the paramedics – an admission directly to the nearest secure psychiatric in-patient unit. Our registrar colleague reported that, over the weekend, she and the nursing staff had observed some worrying signs: incoherence in speech that sounded more like delirium than 'thought disorder', intermittent visual hallucinations (of tiny human beings) interspersed with much more calm and reasonable periods. The registrar employed her excellent medical skills and referred the man to a neurology clinic. A scan revealed a bleed from a ruptured aneurism in the frontal lobes of his brain. By the time we arrived on Monday morning for the 'ward round', the young man had already had surgery. Remarkably, by that time he was back to his normal self – coherent and calm. When we met to discuss his experiences, and to tell him that an acute psychiatric ward was the wrong place for him, he was one of the most content residents on the ward.

It is probably not too surprising that '...an acute psychiatric ward was probably the wrong place for him....' But that tells us something. These kinds of medical emergencies are very rare. It is, of course, hugely important that they are spotted and addressed. I should make it clear: in any residential mental health unit based on a psychosocial ethos, medical advice would be vital. But when such medical emergencies are discovered, it turns out that psychiatric units are exactly the wrong place for people concerned: they need, as in this example, medical or neurological care. Any sensible plans for residential units (in-patient units, as they are currently thought of) should ensure that such medical support is easily available if needed. But it is also important to note how rare examples like this are in reality. The majority of people admitted to psychiatric units are either already well known to ward staff, including the doctors, or have reached the doors of an in-patient unit following a string of contacts with services. In all these contacts – with GPs, with out-patient psychiatrists, with psychologists, social workers and community psychiatric nurses, at Accident and Emergency departments, with the police and with paramedics attached to ambulance services, it is important that, as now, staff are able to identify and refer to medical colleagues anyone who needs their help.

We must identify and respond to critical medical emergencies. Any changes to the design and management of residential, or in-patient, provision must address this issue. But this is only a very rare, very niche, element of the present psychiatric in-patient system. In truth, such medical emergencies are rare. And high quality medical care can be provided in a range of settings. Indeed, there are good reasons to believe that different arrangements may be beneficial.

In our current system, the physical health of residents in in-patient psychiatric wards is a matter for concern. A report in 2012 from the Royal College of Psychiatrists and the Healthcare Quality Improvement Partnership attempted to audit the 'in-patient' care offered to people who had received a diagnosis of 'schizophrenia'.[2] Part of their report addressed physical healthcare needs, and in particular examined the extent to which services met the specific requirements of the NICE clinical guidelines for 'schizophrenia'. These guidelines are not legally binding, but they do represent the standards against which services are audited. The NICE clinical guideline for the care of people with a diagnosis of 'schizophrenia' sets out (in 'standard 4') eight indicators against which physical health should be monitored. These include: body mass index (BMI), blood levels of glucose and lipids (total cholesterol and other fats), blood pressure, smoking habits, alcohol and other substance use, blood levels of the hormone prolactin (where relevant) and a history of cardiovascular disease, diabetes, hypertension or hyperlipidaemia in members of the service user's family. All of these can be addressed quite simply through a brief interview and a blood test – I was recently offered precisely this service from my GP, a 'men's health check'.

Unfortunately, the 2012 audit revealed some rather poor statistics. Monitoring of BMI, blood glucose and lipid levels and blood pressure was only offered to 50% of people (even those who had been in the service a long time). In some 90% of cases, substance use, alcohol use or smoking status were recorded, but prolactin levels had been recorded for only about 10% of cases. The report concludes that in only 29% of cases were the most important 'cardiometabolic risk parameters' recorded. In other words, these crucial health checks were only infrequently offered.

Service users need high quality medical care for their physical health needs. Unfortunately, our current service structures may not allow psychiatric colleagues to provide it. A 2009 report from the Royal College of Psychiatrists[3] (p. 9) concludes that '... there is a growing body of evidence that many psychiatrists lack the skills required to provide for the general healthcare of people with mental health problems. This situation may have arisen for good reason – psychiatrists have sought to specialise in mental health matters, regarding physical healthcare as the province of other clinicians'. My point is that the present system is failing even to live up to the requirements of a biomedical approach to mental healthcare. Once again, we need something different.

## Social breakdown

I remember another ward round at the same psychiatric intensive care unit. Our client was a middle-aged man whose primary problem at the time of admission was hearing nasty, distressing voices ('auditory hallucinations', in medical language). He had received, inevitably, a diagnosis of 'schizophrenia' several years earlier, was well known to services, and had (more or less) adhered to a prescription for 'anti-psychotic' medication over that time. When we met to discuss his case, we saw a man whose regime of medication seemed appropriate, if ineffective. A lesser clinician may have responded to on-going auditory hallucinations by increasing (dangerously) the man's prescription. Luckily, the psychiatrist with whom I worked was better than that. For a while we discussed possible ways that we might be able to help the man to overcome or eliminate the voices. But then...it occurred to us. This man had lived with his voices for many years. He struggled, and he needed help of various kinds, but for many years he had lived successfully on his own. He had experienced auditory hallucinations for many, many years. More recently, something had gone wrong; his self-care had deteriorated and his problems had escalated. There were, of course, reasons for this deterioration, but that's not my point here. My point is that he had found a way of living successfully despite quite distressing auditory hallucinations, but a deterioration in his social circumstances had led to a crisis requiring an emergency response. It struck us – all – in the 'ward round' that the only reasonable outcome that we could expect in the short term would be for him to be able to return to his apartment, able to live his life in a manner of his choosing, with appropriate support, despite hearing voices. It would be lovely to see him free of them, but his ability to live independently was clearly not dependent on their absence. With that realisation, our care plan changed; instead of trying to remove the voices, instead of assuming that his discharge from hospital would be dependent upon successful reduction in the hallucinations, we aimed to help him return to an ability to live independently.

There are many different stories leading people to end up in hospital. For Jacqui Dillon, the colleague whose story opened this book, the birth of her daughter was the trigger for the return of terrors from her childhood. For a close relative of mine, the trigger for a serious 'relapse' was the withdrawal of benefits. The UK Government has recently initiated a change to the 'Employment and Support Allowance' paid to people unable to work. To receive these payments, claimants have to pass a 'work capability assessment' – a short medical test carried out by a private contractor. Many, including my relative 'fail' this test...and the consequences can be serious. In his case, the resulting anxiety led to a deterioration in his mental health. My point is that it is life events and circumstances that lead people into crisis, and into the need for care. In Chapter 4 I outlined some of the social factors that need to be taken into account as part of a holistic assessment of someone's needs. These indicate, by definition, some of the reasons why people get into difficulty. They include such things as loved ones becoming ill or dying, bullying and abuse, major life events, redundancy and unemployment, financial difficulties and debt, marital problems and loneliness.

When people's lives come crashing down around them, when they lose hope, or lose touch with reality, we need to offer them support. If necessary we should offer them a place to stay, a 'place of safety'. We should offer people those services that might actually address their problems; social services, debt counselling, housing advice, benefits advice, employment support, training and educational opportunities, occupational and psychological therapies, physical healthcare. But none of that means that we need to offer them a place in a 'hospital'. We have examples of what is possible from other areas of social and personal care. Care for people with learning disabilities is often delivered in residential units that are predicated on social rather than medical ideas. Residential care for older adults offers a wide range of specialist services in non-medical settings, and hospices are frequently designed and organised in deliberately non-medical ways. There are government plans for more home-based and non-hospital care.[4] Innovative mental health and social services already operate residential crisis units which are often away from traditional hospital sites and typically cater for people in acute distress and in need of immediate support.

## Where would YOU go in a crisis?

Like most people, I have a view on what I'd like in a hotel. I don't suggest that it is an appropriate use of taxpayers' money to offer all users of mental health services a Maldives chalet by the shores of the Indian Ocean, but I do think it's reasonable to consider what we would look for in a decent hotel. People who are stressed, confused, hopeless and low in self-esteem need to be offered accommodation that is high quality, welcoming, supportive and calm, and where they can receive the help they need. In many ways, like a well-staffed 4-star hotel, rather than an emergency medical facility.

I do not doubt that everybody involved in crisis care aspires to offer high quality and physically attractive accommodation. But I fear that the ethos within which care is offered also plays a role. Within a medical, 'disease-model' ethos, the main function of an in-patient ward is to keep someone safe whilst their underlying 'illness' is diagnosed and treated. Other aspects matter less: the atmosphere, the furnishings, the possibility of privacy, the 'messages' that the physical surroundings give about people's worth and status, even staff attitudes. In a 'health' service, there is always a danger that design considerations will follow from medical ways of thinking. People entering residential, in-patient care are often at their most desperate. Few, if any, will feel good about themselves. How must it feel to walk through 'air-lock' style security doors to enter the ward, to be faced with noisy, crowded, functional rooms with institutional, clinical, utilitarian, often shabby fixtures and fittings? But, on the other hand, what could it do for someone to find themselves in an environment which is bright, calm, welcoming, comfortable, elegant and well designed?

The history of mental health services reveals something curious, however. Throughout history, moral considerations have impinged on the otherwise practical, scientific or medical ways of thinking. Perhaps this isn't too surprising. Our mental health and well-being are intimately related to the framework of understanding that we have about ourselves, other people, the world and the future. They concern who we are and why we do what we do, the meaning and purpose of our behaviour and why our lives have turned out as they have. Most importantly, ideas about mental health are invoked to explain why people behave in ways which are frowned upon socially. So it is perhaps to be expected that moral and even religious perspectives have been important concomitants of understanding, care and treatment. This has meant that people with mental health problems have variously been seen as sinners, morally 'lost', animalistic or diseased. And quite barbaric 'treatments' have been used – chairs that spin people around until they are sick, cold baths, insulin 'shock therapy', electric shock therapy, restraint of various kinds and the use of a wide range of sedating drugs. Punitive 'treatment' seems (unconsciously I hope) to have been designed to shock or even punish people for their temerity in becoming embarrassingly distressed – maybe they even have the gall to complain that they have been abused.

Which all means that many people will feel a historical shudder when I propose offering people the equivalent of 4-star hotel accommodation. We have, I fear, a vestige of these blaming, stigmatising, discriminatory attitudes; an unspoken desire to punish people or to shock them into sanity. My own profession of psychology has been complicit here, not only in looking for people's so-called 'deficits', but also helping design interventions based on 'negative reinforcement' or 'aversive stimuli'. There may be those who object to using taxpayers' money to providing hotel standard accommodation to people who are variously 'unemployed', 'on benefits', 'drug-users', 'mentally-ill'.... A simple reading of the media headlines of recent years tends to suggest that as a society we have some rather unpleasant views about how we should treat people. A proposal that general hospitals should aspire to offer the amenities of a 4-star hotel – for instance that a hospice for people with terminal illnesses should be comfortable, elegant, calm, well-appointed – would be uncontroversial. I suggest that any difference in attitude reflects longstanding stigma and discrimination against those of us who admit to emotional distress. Therefore, yes, we should aspire to high quality residential care, and confront the discriminatory attitudes that argue against this.

Having worked in acute mental health units for most of my professional life, I am well aware that safety and security are important. Most mental health professionals are very keen to preserve their clients' personal, family and home lives, and to maintain people's mental health without resorting to residential care. Therefore, especially these days, admission to residential mental health care tends to be reserved for people in acute crisis. It is an unfortunate fact that, therefore, many people in such establishments are either very vulnerable or pose a degree of risk to themselves. So units need to keep people safe. For example, since some people are likely to be experiencing suicidal feelings, it is important to reduce the risk of suicide by hanging. And one of the best ways to do that is by removing ligature points (things that people could hang themselves from).[5] I am also very aware that people, when frustrated, confused, angry and hurt, occasionally pose a real risk to others.

So residential units for people in crisis need to be secure. That costs money, in design and in staffing. And while good design might cost little, part of the lamentable quality of psychiatric units at present may be due to cost savings. But it is entirely possible to design well and maintain security. Part of my job has involved visiting junior civil servants, and very occasionally, government ministers, in Whitehall. Their offices are elegant, occasionally impressive ... and always very secure. When we design for civil servants and politicians, we manage to combine attractive environments with excellent security. It clearly isn't impossible. There are undoubted challenges in designing high quality, secure, residential units. But I cannot conclude that a medical ethos adds anything positive to the experience of residential care. Ultimately, a reliance on chemical restraints is a bad thing.

## Too much coercion?

In February 2013, my colleague (and former PhD supervisor) Professor Richard Bentall, wrote a short article for the Guardian newspaper on the subject of coercion in mental health services. It is worth reading in full, and coincides closely with my own views.[6] It is also well worth reading a commentary on Richard's article by Dina Poursanidou, a member of the Asylum Collective and someone who can speak from personal experience.[7] In his article, Richard makes reference to the fact that coercion is increasing in mental health services. He points out that coercion is 'routine', with many people who are in hospital on a 'voluntary' basis nevertheless detained in all but name, with it being made clear to them that, if they don't agree to the care that is being offered, they will be detained and forced anyway. Richard points out how important a sense of autonomy – the right to make choices – is for all of us, and therefore how coercion and the denial of rights are traumatic. Given that many people using mental health services have already been subjected to physical and sexual abuse, bullying and other kinds of victimisation, further coercion may be particularly traumatic. As Dina comments, the ward to which she was compulsorily admitted became '...the ultimate symbol of an oppressive, terrifying, non-therapeutic and unsafe space in my psyche, a space that I came to hate and despise vehemently...the ultimate symbol of a deeply traumatising experience....' It had come '...to symbolise the culmination of my mental distress for me – a place where I was deprived of my liberty, where I was treated as somebody with diminished capacity and insight....' Dina comments how involuntary detention '...was a source of profound feelings of humiliation and shame, as well as a source of a deep sense of failure, unfairness/injustice and stigmatisation – all acutely disempowering emotions...it was an immensely scarring experience whereby the very core of my existence was deeply shaken and all my certainties collapsed – something that I experienced as a brutal assault on my identity.' Richard Bentall argues that many of the arguments in favour of compulsion are flawed. People are not always (as is often implied) irrational in rejecting care, the medication that is almost always the first choice for clinicians is not always beneficial, and such care often does not have positive long-term outcomes.

Dina is more powerful, commenting that her experience was one of a '...complete lack of therapeutic care on the ward'. Her comments about what happened in reality are worth reading. Bentall concludes that '...sometimes, coercion is difficult to avoid. But if coercion is a necessary evil it is still an evil and mental health services need to find ways of resorting to it less. This will require a change of culture and, perhaps, for some mental health professionals to consider alternative careers. In the long term, the solution to the problem of coercion in psychiatry is to design services that patients find helpful and actually want to use.'

I agree. That is precisely the thrust of this book. But if coercion – even very occasionally – is a necessary evil, how should we frame and use the law?

## The law

One radical proposal is that the law should be silent on the issue of emotional difficulties. For those of a radical, liberal, tradition who take a psychosocial view of mental health issues, there is no need to consider compulsion. If someone is distressed, their argument goes, they should be able to choose for themselves whether to accept psychiatric (or any other form of) care. In this view, if a person chooses to reject the advice of doctors, for example that they should take medication or come into hospital, then that is their right. In this view, we have no right to compel people to undergo psychiatric care.

Few people accept this argument entirely. I don't accept it. People are – have always been – vulnerable to great distress, confusion and hopelessness. Each year about 6,000 people in the UK and 800,000 across the world take their own lives. I mentioned in Chapter 1 how around 1,000 more people killed themselves in the years between 2008 and 2010 than would have been expected, and that this has been associated with the economic recession. I do not regard these people as suffering from 'disorders', but equally I cannot accept that our proper response should be to offer people in huge distress, and not in their usual or 'right' frame of mind the promise that services are there if they want them and leave them to make their own decisions. It is clear that there are frequently times in our lives when we are unable to make rational decisions.

Compulsory mental health care in the United Kingdom is governed by the Mental Health Act 1983 as recently amended by the Mental Health Act 2007.[8] The Mental Health Act states that it is intended to provide for 'the reception, care and treatment of mentally disordered patients, the management of their property and other related matters' where '"mental disorder" means any disorder or disability of the mind'. This circular language (mental disorder means a disorder of the mind) is very common in legal circles, and I find it personally frustrating. I am no follower of Descartian dualism (the idea, wrong in my opinion, that there is a natural separation between 'mind' and 'brain'), but it is interesting that one of the amendments brought in by the 2007 amendments was to remove the two words '…or brain…' from that definition. The Act has many sections (the origin of the term 'to be sectioned' meaning to be detained in hospital under the provisions of the legislation), but central to most people's experiences are Sections 2 and 3.

Section 2 of the Mental Health Act (as amended) allows for a person to be admitted to hospital – whether or not they consent – for assessment for up to 28 days. The legal procedure is that an 'approved mental health professional' or the person's 'nearest relative' (both of these are legal terms, which are largely self-explanatory, the exact legal details can be found online[9]) can apply for admission via the normal referral routes of the health services. Any admission must be authorised by two doctors, who should both agree that: '...the patient is suffering from a mental disorder of a nature or degree that warrants detention in hospital for assessment; and that the patient ought to be detained for his or her own health or safety, or the protection of others....' In an emergency, a person can be detained for up to 72 hours, if one doctor has confirmed that '...the detention is of "urgent necessity..."' and that '...waiting for a second doctor to approve the detention...would cause an "undesirable delay"'. In addition, as mentioned earlier, police officers have the authority to take people to a 'place of safety' if they appear to be suffering from a mental disorder, in order that they be assessed by a doctor and an approved mental health professional.

Section 3 of the Act is very similar, except that it permits detention in hospital for up to six months, and for the purposes of treatment as well as assessment. In the words of the Act, '...detention can last for up to six months after two doctors have confirmed that the patient is suffering from mental disorder of a nature or degree which makes it appropriate for the patient to receive medical treatment in a hospital, the treatment is in the interests of his or her health and safety and the protection of others and appropriate treatment must be available for the patient.' Of course, some people remain in hospital for longer than this, in some cases for years. Detention under Section 3 can be renewed for a further six months and thereafter for periods of 12 months at a time. Once in hospital, people are under the care of a 'responsible clinician', who – in most cases – will be responsible for deciding when discharge is appropriate.

## A psychosocial perspective

Mental health legislation is a very controversial area. Speaking for myself, but from an informed psychosocial perspective, I do believe that there is a need for such legislation. The powers of the Mental Health Act are used about 50,000 times a year in England and Wales. This does not mean that 50,000 people are detained in hospital, because some people may be detained several times within a year. With very few exceptions, all professionals working in mental health services are very well aware of the serious threat to civil liberties and human rights that this entails, and the frequent trauma that ensues for the individuals involved. My colleagues (or, at least, all those whom I admire) therefore only use the

Act when they believe it to be necessary and in the best interests of their clients. For me, this means two things. First: while there is very wide-spread acceptance that we should try to reduce the number of people subject to compulsion under mental health legislation, there is no set figure – 25,000 or 10,000, say, that is agreed to be the 'correct' figure. Second: the driving force behind our use of compulsion in mental health care is necessity – the idea that some people need urgent help, and that we cannot, in conscience, abandon them. Nevertheless, in my opinion, significant revisions of the UK's mental health legislation are required. These can learn from, and possibly inform, other jurisdictions' approaches.

The present UK Mental Health Act is, like many other national vari-ants, a very odd piece of legislation. It almost elides the central issue: it slips past the point. In any normal state of affairs, it would clearly be illegal – a form of unlawful imprisonment – to require someone to stay in hospital if they wished to leave, and equally illegal – a form of assault – to force a person to take medication if they did not consent. Clearly, these things are not illegal if performed under the auspices of the Mental Health Act and if the required conditions are met. I hinted earlier at Section 136 powers, which enable a police officer to take someone whom they believe to be 'mentally disordered' from a public place to a 'place of safety'. Interestingly, if the person is in a private place, the Act (in Section 135) requires a police officer first to obtain a warrant from a magistrate (junior judge). And that contrast illustrates how the Mental Health Act is a permissive Act – it permits people to do things that would otherwise be illegal or require a warrant.

And the things it permits are serious. If deployed incorrectly, use of mental health legislation could lead to serious breaches of human rights. Article 3 of the European Convention on Human Rights (and therefore of the UK Human Rights Act 1998) states that 'no one shall be subjected to torture or to inhuman or degrading treatment or punish-ment'. Many of us would argue that much of current mental health care is perceived by a very large number of people to be degrading and inhu-mane. Indeed, the unusual American techniques used to modify the behaviour of children with 'autistic' problems that I mentioned in the introductory chapter were actually described as 'akin to torture'. Article 5 states that 'everyone has the right to liberty and security of person. No one shall be deprived of his liberty save in the following cases and in accordance with a procedure prescribed by law....' One of these 'cases' concerns 'the lawful detention of ... persons of unsound mind...'. The term 'of unsound mind' is not defined in the Human Rights Act, but case law has referred to people with 'real illnesses'.[10] Obviously, given the discussions in Chapter 2 of this book, I reject the notion of 'real illnesses'. To be clear, not only do I believe that there are no such things as 'real mental illnesses', I believe the notion is irrelevant. If we were to accept, for the point of argument, that a 'real mental illness' were to be defined as 'meeting the criteria for a recognised mental illness as defined by one of the major diagnostic manuals', clearly this would not render a person liable to mental health legislation – caffeine dependence and trichotillomania (hair pulling) are 'recognised mental disorders' in those manuals, and nobody would suggest the Mental Health Act could be used in such cases. In short, I do not believe people are 'ill' and I do not believe they need 'treatment' in a 'hospital'.

But I do believe that some people need help. Under what circumstances should we be permitted to override a person's right to liberty, to be able to choose for themselves where they reside and whether or not to accept professional advice? Article 8 of the European Convention on Human Rights affirms that 'everyone has the right to respect for his private and family life, his home and his correspondence' and 'there shall be no interference by a public authority with the exercise of this right except such as is in accordance with the law and is necessary in a democratic society in the interests of national security, public safety or the economic well-being of the country, for the prevention of disorder or crime, for the protection of health or morals, or for the protection of the rights and freedoms of others.' Article 8 therefore is also of key importance in the context of compulsory mental health care. It provides for compulsion in the case of necessity.

In my opinion, it is right that the criteria include the requirement to the effect that 'the person is experiencing mental health problems of a nature or degree which makes it appropriate for them to be admitted to a residential care establishment.' I also believe that it is appropriate to include a criterion to the effect that 'it is necessary for the person's health or safety or for the protection of other persons that they should be admitted to a residential care establishment.' These essentially reflect key criteria already in the Mental Health Act of England and Wales. They reflect the serious and compassionate judgement shown by colleagues as they implement the Act. But the English and Welsh Act does not include a further vital criterion. It does not include any reference to the person's ability to make decisions for themselves.

In a psychological approach, a concept such as 'of unsound mind' would only make sense if a person were unable to make valid decisions for themselves. This, vital, extra criterion is absent from the English and Welsh Mental Health Act. Scotland, famously, is a separate nation, with a separate legal system. In Scotland, the Mental Health (Care and Treatment) (Scotland) Act, 2003,[11] includes a criterion 'that because of the mental disorder the patient's ability to make decisions about the provision of such medical treatment is significantly impaired'. In Canada the relevant criteria include that 'the person is unable to understand and to make an informed decision regarding his or her need for treatment, care or supervision as a result of the mental disorder.'

Were English and Welsh law to adopt this criterion, it would draw mental health legislation much closer to the UK's Mental Capacity Act. The Mental Capacity Act is designed to protect people who may permanently or temporarily not be able ('lack capacity') to make some decisions for themselves. The Act covers issues such as 'Enduring Power of Attorney' and is designed to deal with important decisions relating to an individual's property, financial affairs, and health and social care. It also applies to everyday decisions, such as personal care, what to wear and what to eat. It sets out tests for such decision-making capacity and sets out how people may make decisions for people in those circumstances – bearing in mind the legal responsibility to ensure that any decision made on their behalf is made in their best interests. There are obvious points of similarity between the Mental Capacity Act and proposed revisions to the Mental Health Act.

Until recently, compulsory mental health care was very largely restricted to in-patient hospital settings. But discharge has always been a matter of concern. In the UK, clinicians had been in the practice of occasionally offering people 'long leave' – retaining the element of compulsion because the individual was officially 'detained in hospital' but discharged 'on leave'. This practice was ruled unlawful, and in 2007 the UK Government introduced 'community treatment orders'. These allow people to be discharged from hospital, but they are required to adhere to a care plan drawn up by their 'responsible clinician'. Clearly, I have little faith in the benefits of long-term medication, and I passionately support the principle of autonomy for people able to exercise it. But equally I don't think that people are 'ill', and I don't believe in the concept of 'hospital care' in this context. Many mental health problems are not only serious but also longstanding or recurrent. If someone requires on-going help, it may be a 'least restrictive alternative' to supervise people in their own homes. I do think, therefore, that there are circumstances where it might be reasonable to see mental health legislation outside a hospital setting. But it should always be the case that the same principles – necessity and lack of capacity – should guide its use. Importantly, I also believe there should be much greater judicial oversight.

## Warrants

In my opinion, a further change to the law is required. The deprivation of rights and liberties represented by the use of mental health legislation is serious. Although I believe it is reasonable – even necessary – that we care for someone if they are temporarily or permanently unable to exercise rational autonomy, it is important that we have proper judicial oversight over this process. Other intrusions into peoples' rights and liberties are governed by the strict application of warrants, only under exceptional circumstances do we tolerate a 'permissive' approach, merely allowing authorities to override our rights. We (at least in the UK) require a judicial warrant to arrest someone (an 'arrest warrant') or to search someone's house (a 'search warrant'). These aren't particularly difficult to obtain; a police officer makes an application to a duty magistrate, presents evidence that the necessary criteria are met, and the process is sanctioned. Importantly, sanctioned under legal authority. I believe that all applications of mental health legislation – in England and Wales, the Mental Health Act – should be sanctioned by warrant. That would, necessarily, put a hurdle in the process of 'sectioning'. That is right and proper. It is simply appropriate that such a serious legal, as well as clinical, decision should be legally sanctioned. And any pressure to reduce the level of compulsion in mental healthcare should be welcomed. Most importantly, it is right that evidence that someone meets the criteria for the legislation to be applied – including that they are not able to exercise their own decision, making autonomy at that point – is presented to a neutral, judicial person before action is taken.

In my opinion, then, we should only use the savage powers of mental health legislation when a magistrate or judge has issued a warrant after first being persuaded both that detention is necessary for the person's health or safety or that of others, and also that the person is unable at that point to make an informed decision regarding their care. This would certainly not mean that a person in great and acute distress (and, perhaps, causing a public disturbance) would be left without help while complex bureaucratic processes are pursued to obtain a warrant. It is clearly important to balance a desire for judicial oversight with a need for urgent action to assist people in distress. As with arrest or search warrants in the criminal justice system, however, it is perfectly possible to legislate for a reasonable balance in these issues. The various sections of the UK's Mental Health Act already include provisions for immediate response to acute need, with subsequent actions required within 72 hours. What would differ if there were proper judicial review is that, within 72 hours, a warrant would be required from the courts. This is different from the present system that merely requires compliance with the provisions of the legislation without specific judicial oversight.

## Psychologists and compulsion

Until recently, psychologists have not been directly involved in imposing compulsory mental health care. In England and Wales, the amendments to the Mental Health Act in 2007 brought a significant change in the form of the new role of 'responsible clinician'. The 'responsible clinician' replaces the old role of 'responsible medical officer' and is the person responsible for a person's care while detained under the Mental Health Act. Clinical Psychologists as well as psychiatrists can now be 'responsible clinicians'. This is a profound change in our potential role within mental health care (although, of course, it will apply to those of us who adopt this responsibility). Indeed, the psychologist David Smail has said: 'what makes [psychologists] different from other professions in the field is ... [that we] ... can't lock them up; we can't drug them or stun them with electricity; we can't take their children away from them. The only power we have is the power of persuasion and this ... more or less forces us into an attitude of respect towards our clients'.[12] Clearly, this relationship between clinical psychologists and their clients could be threatened by compulsion. But, in my opinion, what makes psychologists different from other professions is not only a historical absence of formal power but also a markedly different framework of knowledge and skills. The argument made in this book is that a different, new psychosocial model of care is required. Although I am well aware of the potential dangers, I am also of the opinion that this different approach to care planning should be available – should particularly be available – to people in the most acute need. In time, I believe it should be routine for the 'responsible clinician' to be a psychologist or social worker.

# 6
# Teamworking

*Services should be equipped to address the full range of people's social, personal and psychological as well as medical needs. Teams should be multidisciplinary, democratic and aligned to a psychosocial model. This would involve a greater reliance on psychological therapies, and suggests that many nursing and medical colleagues should consider retraining. This model also implies a new role for consultant psychiatrists: as expert colleagues, but with leadership of multidisciplinary teams determined by the skills and personal qualities of the individual members of the team. In a psychosocial model of mental health and well-being, there would be no assumption that medical psychiatrists would retain their current authority and status.*

A genuinely psychosocial approach to service delivery would mean increased investment in the full range of professionals able to deliver therapeutic services that address people's genuine problems and their root causes. The service would offer help with a spectrum of psychological difficulties rather than only those deemed 'mental health problems'. Nobody would be 'diagnosed'. There would be a major emphasis on prevention. We need to be able to address such issues as divorce, marital difficulties, unemployment, stresses at work, financial difficulties, illnesses in family members, crime (both as a victim and as a perpetrator, when caught up in the criminal justice system), assaults, bullying, and childhood abuse. Clearly we need to offer psychological therapies, because we know that the way that people make sense of and respond to events is important, and the opportunity to talk through what has happened and how it has affected us is vital. But we also need to offer much more practical responses. As Anne Cooke put it: 'It's no good just mopping the floor and leaving the tap running'. So mental health and well-being services should need to work with the criminal justice agencies to ensure both protection and justice – investigating and preventing assaults. Because marital separation is a major source of emotional stress, we should ensure that there is sufficient support for people going through separation or marital difficulties, such as mediation services, support for single parents, and practical, legal and emotional support for people in difficulty in their relationships. Because unemployment is a major source of distress, we should aim for full employment, and certainly do what we can to protect people from the emotional and economic impact of unemployment. Many jobs are themselves sources of stress, however. We should aim to ensure equitable and supportive employment practices, including employee relations, a living wage, decent terms and conditions and appropriate employee representation. We should engage with employers to address workplace stresses and offer people who are out of work practical, as well as emotional support. Services such as Citizens Advice, debt counselling agencies and Victim Support are vital to help people in financial difficulties, victims of crime and people dealing with a range of other traumatic life events. We should ensure that any mental health and well-being services are fully integrated with other social services that support families and parents in difficulty. It also means working with teachers and educational psychologists in schools, and it means supporting a network of children's services. We should not only offer emotional support, and counsel people in financial difficulties, we should also offer people practical help and financial advice. We should support people in negotiations with benefits agencies to ensure people have the financial support that they deserve, and we should be prepared to engage with financial systems (such as 'pay-day loan' companies) that conspire to keep people indebted. Recreational street drugs can prove a threat to people's mental health and well-being, and so we should ensure that mental health services have intimate links to services that help people who have problems with drug use. Clearly, providing these services properly will entail significant change. Many of these issues are currently largely ignored, and most are ill-coordinated. Apologists for the present systems will argue that all these services are currently part of the care offered to clients. The experiences of those who have passed through the system would tend to suggest otherwise.

The adoption of a 'psychobiosocial' model for the provision of services would have significant implications, as colleagues and I have contended for a while.[1] As I have argued throughout this book, services would be planned on the basis of need and helping people find 'real-world' solutions that work for them, rather than providing 'treatments' according to diagnostic categories. Where residential care is necessary, completely new residential units, operating according to wholly different rules would replace 'hospitals'. This would mean that services would fully embrace the recovery approach; people would not be 'treated' for 'illnesses', but would be helped to regain a better quality of life. The people who use, or have used, the services would be intimately involved in their development and management as well as in the actual provision, with 'expertise by experience' highly valued. The therapies, interventions and services would be guided by individual formulations drawn up collaboratively between the service user and the professionals involved.

In such an approach, there would continue to be an emphasis on specialist teams, but they would be planned and organised on the basis of psychosocial rather than medical principles. As a psychologist, I am naturally likely to argue this, but psychologists should be prepared to offer consultation and clinical leadership. Medicine would remain a key profession, but with emphasis placed on a return to the key principles of applying medical expertise as it assists a multidisciplinary team in the understanding of someone's problems and offering help, rather than on an unquestioned assumption that doctors should lead clinical teams. Nurses should diversify from attending to the medical treatments prescribed by doctors, and develop increasing competencies in psychosocial interventions. Occupational therapists and social workers should see their roles develop and strengthen. We should be open to new possibilities; it would be particularly valuable to employ people skilled in practical issues such as finding employment or training, managing finances and caring for children. Finally, we should see the increased and explicit employment of peer professionals, people with lived experience of mental health problems. Personal experience of mental health problems should even actively be seen as a desirable characteristic in colleagues, rather than an exclusion criterion.

## Access to and provision of services

Decisions about the provision of mental healthcare should be based on individuals' distress and their personal and social functioning, rather than diagnosis of illness. Given the huge impact of mental health problems discussed earlier, there are good arguments for a substantial increase in funding for mental health care. Nevertheless, difficult decisions have to be made about to whom and in what circumstances services should be made available. As I have made clear, any diagnostic distinction between 'real illnesses' and 'normal reactions' is alien to psychological models of mental well-being. Instead, priorities should be based on the severity of, consequences of, and risk posed by a person's problems.

To people who unquestioningly accept the spurious quasi-certainties of a medical diagnostic approach, where you would expect a service if you are 'ill' and not if you aren't, this may appear to be a loose and vague arrangement. But the assessment of psychological difficulties can be conducted on alternative bases that are at least as reliable as diagnosis,[2] and have the major advantage of what scientists call 'ecological validity' – they actually make sense in the real world.[3] In fact, the use of what is called 'stepped care' in the IAPT programme (see Chapter 5) supports this, in that access to different 'steps' or 'stages' is dependent not on diagnosis but on the nature and severity of a person's problems.

## Teams, multidisciplinary teams and democratic multidisciplinary teams

Planning care should be a team-based activity. Clients referred to mental health and well-being services, whether seeing an individual therapist, attending alternative day services or admitted to residential care, should expect to have their full range of relevant needs assessed and then addressed by an appropriate range of properly qualified specialists. As I mentioned in my introductory chapter, the joint UK Department of Health and Royal College of Psychiatrists' 'New Ways of Working' report argued that proper care for people in deep personal distress was a team effort; a multi-professional effort. As I have made clear throughout this book, the range of needs – social, psychological and medical (in different proportions for different people) – means that the team would require a range of specialists working together. In this model, as I argued in my introduction, the nature of extreme distress means that medical colleagues may well be valuable members of the team but they should be consultants *to* the team rather than having sapiential authority *over* it.

The word 'sapiential' was new to me, too. I was involved in the discussions surrounding the New Ways of Working report. One of our tasks was to look at the specific and distinctive contribution that each profession makes to a multidisciplinary team. We received a draft of the working party looking at the distinctive contribution of the consultant psychiatrist. In part, the document acknowledged that; '...a well functioning multi-disciplinary team requires leadership from several individuals with different levels of expertise in different areas – leading on what each knows best...'. But it went on, immediately, to suggest; '...such is the clinical primacy of the consultant in dealing with treatment resistant, acute, severe or dangerous clinical situations that require the broadest possible approach covering all physical, legal, psychological, and social aspects, as well as analysing and making explicit the value and ethical aspects of choices or decisions to be made. It is more sapiential than hierarchical leadership. This will become much clearer with the shift from delegated to distributed responsibility for patients in community mental health teams. It will be up to the autonomous professional to decide when to seek advice or case review with a consultant. And every time that happens it will give meaning to the clinical primacy of the consultant with whom the 'buck stops' in given situations'. In other words...teams need a range of skills, but the consultant psychiatrist should always be in charge. Deconstructing the language used is important. 'Clinical primacy of the consultant' is a phrase that implies a medical professional should be in charge, directly contradicting the immediately preceding statement. This point becomes even clearer when the text suggests that 'the autonomous professional' should seek review from a consultant...with whom the 'buck stops'. So much for autonomy! I, of course, had serious objections to this suggestion. But I was also intrigued by the use of the word sapiential. I had to look it up. The dictionary definition is: 'relating to wisdom'. Most dictionaries add that the word is 'from ecclesiastical Latin' and relates particularly to the wisdom of God.

Well...I disagree. Specifically, I agree that: ' ...a well functioning multidisciplinary team requires leadership from several individuals with different levels of expertise in different areas – leading on what each knows best...'. I do not agree with the concept of 'clinical primacy' and I do not believe that any one profession has 'sapiential leadership'. This draft does not feature in the final report.

The right place for mental health care is in the community – alongside GPs, public health physicians and social workers. There should be a network of community-based care teams, linked to social services provision and other local authority care and services, as well as to the NHS and third-sector organisations. In the UK, at least, this is consistent with a general intention to integrate mental health care, physical health care and social care. We've seen a major integration of GP services with wider community and social services. Importantly, we've recently seen UK public health services transferred wholesale into local authority management. This offers a precedent and a model for similar transfer of responsibilities for mental health care. This vision would see opportunities for GPs, properly trained in mental health care, to help support people's well-being. It would obviously see many more clinical psychologists … But, as with our medical colleagues, they would be working in the community, not in hospitals or 'clinics'. As mentioned earlier, medical psychiatrists would be consultants to, not in charge of, those teams. I envisage psychology-led teams (with an appropriate mix of staff), not psychiatrist-led teams with medical and nursing colleagues.

One of my colleagues, a senior and respected psychiatrist (whom I think it would be unwise and unhelpful to name), recently told me: ' … I think you can make a perfectly coherent argument for the total dissolution of psychiatry. In an ideal world, I don't think it would exist, or if it did, it would simply be medical professionals interested in the care of the mad alongside other professionals, much as it started out being in the asylum days of the 19th century … '. I tend largely to agree. Since our mental health and well-being is predominantly a social and psychological phenomenon, since diagnosis is unhelpful and the prescription of drugs should be reserved for a minority, we should see a much greater reliance on GPs to provide for the holistic healthcare of their patients. In this vision, medical psychiatrists would still perhaps have roles: as specialists, as consultants to GPs and as consultants to residential units. But we should see a major rebalancing of investment away from what is now traditional psychiatry towards a different system. Perhaps not the 'total dissolution of psychiatry', but a very significant change.

## Psychologists

For my chosen profession of clinical psychology, adopting this vision could have significant consequences. Clinical psychology is a profession that has its roots in mental health, and it is highly likely that addressing mental health problems will remain the key focus of our work for the foreseeable future. Clinical psychologists are obviously experts in psychological therapies (or, in the UK at least, must be competent in at least two forms of psychological therapy in order to retain their professional registration with the Health and Care Professions Council), so it is highly likely that we will continue to offer one-to-one therapy. But as well as merely providing therapy, clinical psychologists have been calling for more socially responsible, more fully holistic, services for many years. In practice that would mean a great deal more work across all the domains of well-being discussed earlier. That means linking with employment advisors in JobCentrePlus (the UK Government-run employment and benefits agency) and other occupational health and occupational psychology services – helping people reduce workplace stress, minimising the likelihood of absence due to emotional problems and maximising productivity. It means working with schools and teachers – helping children learn, but also helping children, teachers and parents deal more effectively with emotional issues. In the model for psychosocial mental health and well-being services I am discussing here, we would expect to see clinical psychologists working more closely with the physical health services – supporting patients with serious physical illnesses, helping them adjust to illness or injury, helping with rehabilitation, maximising the likelihood that people take steps towards becoming fitter and healthier. Across a wide range of community services we should see clinical psychologists offering their skills in sports and leisure, with charities, with local authority services... across the full breadth of the domains of well-being.

To achieve that, our employers need to understand – and support – this move. Most clinical psychologists in the UK are currently employed by NHS Trusts. It is perhaps unfortunate that our history of close links with mental health services, and our undoubted expertise in one-to-one psychological therapies, mean that clinical psychologists are often seen as valued staff if and when they see individual clients, but are less often encouraged to pursue these broader roles. As I have made clear already but will expand upon in the next chapter, I believe it would be better if mental health services as a whole, including clinical psychologists, were managed in local authority settings. There could be many benefits for my profession.

A focus beyond 'mental health', or, worse 'mental illness', and instead addressing well-being more broadly would mean looking at our links with the other applied psychologist groups. A genuine view of well-being integrates clinical psychologists' interest in mental health with occupational psychologists' interest in employment, educational psychologists' interest in education, health psychologists, forensic psychologists and so on. All these professional groups apply our knowledge of psychological theory to addressing social problems and improving well-being. So this is less a call for clinical psychologists as a very specific group to broaden their ambitions across all of life, but rather more a call for applied psychologists to work together to apply their skills and knowledge in a coherent manner across all these domains of well-being. In my opinion, we should be bold. I believe that applied psychology itself needs to reform. We need to unify our currently disparate 'brands' of applied psychology into a single profession – and we need to make that profession more genuinely fit for purpose. That means looking at our professional body, the British Psychological Society, and reforming it

such that it more closely resembles other Royal Colleges and representa-
tive professional bodies. It would also mean looking at our training. In a
paper published in 2002 that was a few years ahead of its time, I recommended that one way to make our profession more suited to the model
of mental health and well-being discussed here might be to have more
integration in our training.[4] I recommended that we should consider
training occupational, clinical, health, educational and forensic psychologists together in a generic curriculum in the first year of our three-year
doctoral training, tapering to specialist training in year three. I argued
that this approach would retain specialist training through the tapered
specialisation. This would ensure that each person would finish their
training with the skills necessary to register as a clinical or occupational
psychologist or indeed in any other branch of applied psychology, rather
than have to adopt the rather vague and over-general term of 'applied
psychologist'. The benefit of the scheme is that each person would have
pursued a pathway through training that will have involved a much
greater degree of integrated exposure to other approaches within applied
psychology. That, clearly, would render applied psychology and hence
clinical psychology, better equipped for the design of services I hope we
will be able to adopt.

## Social workers

There are powerful arguments to suggest that the most appropriate professionals to coordinate such services should be social workers. My argument
throughout this book has been that people's emotional distress is largely
determined by their social circumstances and life events. It makes sense,
then, to see mental health and well-being services as integral to the social
services delivered (in the UK) by local authorities. As I have – I hope –
made clear, I not only see the future of mental health and well-being
services as lying within those wider social services, and indeed organised and managed through local authorities, but I envisage a much more
'social' ethos behind those services. Meaningful recovery – defined in
terms of social, psychological or occupational functioning – is influenced
as much by social class, opportunities for employment and economic
and social policy as by 'successful' treatment of what we currently think
of as psychiatric symptoms.[5] Social factors should therefore be integrated with psychological and biological elements in any care plan, and
social interventions strongly supported. Social workers are currently the
only mental health workers with specific and comprehensive education and training in social science.[6] The training of social workers – like

psychologists, psychiatrists and nurses – covers a wide range of theoretical perspectives and skills. The distinctive contribution of social workers, perhaps especially in promoting social inclusion, means they have important roles in organising and commissioning care packages beyond the NHS. While this is valuable, it may be worth considering the slightly more direct and therapeutic role offered by 'social pedagogues' elsewhere in the EU.[7] This is a professional approach with a particular focus on early years education, but which can be useful with any age group. Not unlike occupational therapists, social pedagogues deploy a wide range of academic disciplines (sociology, psychology, education, philosophy, the medical sciences and social work) to help people develop their skills and self confidence in dealing with emotions and relationships.

## Psychiatry

Psychiatrists have an important role in any multidisciplinary mental health and well-being service, but might be well advised to better refocus their efforts on medical healthcare and on the specifically biological aspects of mental health. This would mean a more specific focus on physical health (although, as I shall explain later, family doctors or GPs would be more appropriate for this purpose for most people), including identifying those very rare cases where a person's apparent psychological problems have a physical cause, as in the aneurysm example above (although such cases are rare, it is important to provide this service) and on the prescription of psychiatric drugs (although, as I have made clear, I would wish to see a sharply reduced reliance on such medication). I have discussed both these elements in detail elsewhere in this book. I have made it clear how both are important, and how both are, in fact, inadequate in the current configuration of services. I believe that physical healthcare requires close liaison with community-based, primary care healthcare systems (in the UK, the GPs who offer our comprehensive first point of care and family doctor services). It is also important that mental health services have competent medical professionals to assess the possible contribution of biological causative factors to mental health and prescribe drugs (if people want to take them). So psychiatrists and other medical staff would remain a crucial component of care.

## Nursing

With profound changes in the use of medical staff, there could be significant changes to the role of nurses. In the UK, mental health nurses form the backbone of services, acting as frontline carers, and commonly offer 24 hours a day, 7 days a week care. There are over 45,000 mental health nurses in the UK.[8] This reflects the fact that mental health nurses work in all areas of mental health services, and frequently act as care coordinators. For many people, nurses are the only direct care providers, although their role is increasingly being taken over by unqualified 'support workers'. Their extended and close contact with service users means that it is often only a nurse that has a detailed knowledge of the individual, their carers and families. In the psychosocial vision I am offering, mental health nurses could further develop competencies in psychosocial interventions.[9] The model of service provision I am proposing would support the development of the autonomy and independence of nurses in a 'consultant' role, and strongly support the development of nurses' competencies in psychological aspects of care and in psychological interventions. In recent years, the role of the mental health nurse has already evolved in this direction, but there is a convincing argument for a substantial change in the nature and profile of the nursing role. I believe that the training of 'nurses' should reflect the science of mental health care; and should stress psychosocial, not medical interventions. I would much prefer to offer my colleagues training in new approaches rather than to argue that we should replace them. We should even consider changing the name of the profession to reflect its new emphasis. The 'nurse' role and title again stem from healthcare, from medicine and could be argued to be inappropriate in a psychosocial service. Although likely to be controversial, renaming 'nurses' might be a very powerful way to signal change in the system. Of course, it would be for my colleagues to define their own identity, but a possibility would be something like 'psychosocial therapist'.

## Occupational therapists

Most people would expect – hope – that purposeful activity would be an important element of all forms of mental health care. This is true both in community settings and in residential care. I quoted a short extract from a letter I had received in the introductory chapter, from a man describing his experiences on a psychiatric inpatient ward. This is not at all what residential units should be like. It may indeed be a fantasy, but I can imagine a world in which a day spent in a residential mental health unit would involve practical steps towards health in the form of physical exercise – a trip to a gym or to a swimming pool, perhaps – and purposeful activity during the day; activity that is therapeutic, is geared towards the 'five ways to well-being' and is meaningful to each person. I simply don't think that is too much to ask for.

Work is known to be important in promoting recovery for those who have experienced mental health problems[10] but people face major challenges in the employment market.[11] Occupational therapy addresses 'the nature, balance, pattern and context of occupations and activities in the lives of individuals, family groups and communities'[12] but occupational therapists, like other professions, are also rapidly developing skills in psychological therapies. Like social workers, occupational therapists also have a particular focus on issues of social inclusion, with many people reporting a dearth of meaningful, therapeutic, purposeful activity in mental health care; something many people equate to an over-reliance on medical approaches. Occupational therapy – again perhaps with a more appropriate name, and again perhaps with shades of 'social pedagogy' – should be central to psychosocial services.

## What's new?

Many commentators, many critics, would no doubt say that this (or perhaps elements of this) are happening already. They might point to the fact that a number of government initiatives have supported psychosocial approaches, have emphasised patient-centred services, supported a 'recovery' approach and, of course, the UK Government has launched the IAPT – improving access to psychological therapies – programme. They would argue that developments such as 'New Ways of Working' have repeatedly stressed the importance of multidisciplinary teams, and of a biopsychosocial model underpinning care. Most importantly they would point to the inclusion of such services as debt counselling, drugs services, court diversion schemes and the creative arts of various kinds in the 'landscape of care'. Many people would applaud the suggestion that mental health services should link 'more closely with grass-roots voluntary agencies and self-help groups, including offering helping-the-helpers support, or taking responsibility ourselves for training and supervising community members'.[13] But, positive though all these developments are, in my view they fail to address the main problem. Worse, by failing to challenge the 'disease model' of mental health, they leave intact the basic, damaging, idea that currently drives our mental health services, namely that psychological and emotional difficulties are merely symptoms of an underlying physical 'mental illness', a brains disease. For many of my colleagues promoting a more humane approach, half-hearted claims to be addressing social issues (often, as is implicit in the quotation above, through *somebody else*'s services) threaten to render arguments for change impotent. The real change that we so badly need will only come when we move beyond the idea that mental health issues are essentially a medical problem with social aspects, and acknowledge that what we are talking about are essentially social problems. Radical change is needed to ensure that the management, leadership and practices of services reflect this.

# 7
# Social and Community Services in Local Authority Management

*Mental health services should be based in local authorities, alongside other social, community-based, services. The psychological, emotional and behavioural problems that are commonly referred to as mental health problems are fundamentally social and psychological issues rather than medical illnesses. It follows that the correct place for services to support mental health and well-being is within the social care system. We should, to be clear, go further than design what are essentially medical teams for psychiatry, managed as out-patient hospital-based teams. Instead, mental health and well-being teams should be part of community social services, and therefore under local authority control. The recent transfer of UK public health services to local authority control is a positive example of this approach in practice.*

The thrust of the arguments in this book culminates in a simple message. The psychological, emotional and behavioural problems that are commonly referred to as mental health problems are fundamentally social and psychological issues. Psychologists, therapists and social workers must work closely alongside GPs, public health physicians and nurses. But mental health and well-being is fundamentally a psychological and social phenomenon, with medical aspects. It is not, fundamentally, a medical phenomenon with additional psychological and social elements. It follows that the correct place for mental health care is within the social care system. That doesn't mean that we should design medical teams for psychiatry, and manage them out of hospital-based, NHS-based trusts but housed in a building away from the hospital site as a gesture towards being 'community-based'. Instead, it means that we should locate the whole service in the community – put it entirely under local authority control. In the UK, we have the model of public health, recently transferred to local authority control, to build upon. Such services should be – and could then be – under democratic local governance.

Change is needed, because the present system places care for people with psychological problems – so-called 'mental health' care – in a medical context. In many ways, this is an unhappy relationship. As with public health (an example to which I shall return), complicated and unusual arrangements need to be put in place in order to ensure that we can meet people's very real social and psychological needs, which do not always fit well within a medical model. The fundamental 'mission statement' of a medical healthcare system is very different to that of a system for social care and support. In the first, leadership, even dominance, by medical practitioners is natural, and medical assumptions pervade the system. The 'disease-model' and 'diagnosis-treat' approach, the assumption that we are dealing with 'syndromes', 'illnesses' and 'pathology' are all taken for granted. In many ways, the structures within which mental health care is currently located are part of the problem. We can imagine a service in which problems are identified and solutions developed without any need for assumptions of 'illness' and 'pathology'. But it is difficult to imagine that service operating easily within a wider, overarching system that remains reliant on precisely those inappropriate assumptions.

I once attended a rather odd meeting of a range of senior 'mental health' professionals. It was odd because it was arranged over dinner…which led to people being quite informal in their conversation. Towards the end of the meeting, one of the participants, a very senior psychiatrist, tried to sum up the emerging friendly consensus by saying: 'ultimately we all have the same aim – we're all in the business of treating illnesses…'. I disagree…and said so. That simply does not sum up my role as a clinical psychologist. I do not think that I am 'in the business of treating illnesses'. My business is using my knowledge of psychology to help people improve their psychological and emotional well-being and to solve difficult problems in their lives. That is not the same as 'treating illnesses'. I recognise that psychiatry and nursing, because they are professions related to medicine, are happier within that role. But the concept of 'treating illness' is a wholly inappropriate basis for a consensus – because it simply fails to reflect non-medical perspectives. It is also an inappropriate model for our service more generally. In my view it is inappropriate to regard people as 'ill'. But this kind of casual language use reflects a mistaken assumption about the ethos and character of a nationwide service employing many thousands of dedicated professionals. Many of these professionals understand their clients' – and indeed their own – emotional lives very differently. This kind of language also reflects the dominant mode of operation in our current structures for delivering care. A fundamental shift is needed.

## Social agents in a social model

In my vision of mental health care, we should act primarily as social agents in a social model of care. The best system for organising and delivering this care would therefore be through the social services of the local authorities. In the UK this would see what is now considered part of the NHS, the health care system, becoming part of the local authority Social Services provision. In other countries, the systems for provision are slightly different, but the basic separation of social and medical care is commonplace. The transfer of responsibilities that I am suggesting may, in fact, be somewhat easier in other countries than in the UK, because city and regional authorities often have responsibilities for healthcare, which in the UK is organised on a quasi-national basis.

Let's take a concrete example: the city in which I work, Liverpool in North West England. I would like to see Liverpool City Council take over responsibility for the strategic direction, management and delivery of mental health care for the city. In this vision, all the mental health care – the services that are now delivered through health services structures such as NHS trusts – would be managed and delivered by local authorities. This would see psychiatry and associated professions organised and managed alongside existing social services and the public health colleagues who have already been brought under local authority management. Of course, at present, much of our mental health care is already delivered in community settings. But it remains part of, and organised by, the National Health Service. And residential care in particular remains dominated by hospital-based in-patient psychiatric wards. A more appropriate model would be for mental health to be based entirely within local social services. That would mean seeing local authorities assuming management of the whole system, including residential or 'in-patient' units. And those in-patient wards would be re-configured as residential units along social, not medical, lines. This would be a fundamental change.

Psychiatry as a profession is a branch of medicine – psychiatrists are medical practitioners, members of the British Medical Association, regulated by the General Medical Council and organised into a Royal College. As psychiatry is de facto the dominant profession in mental healthcare, much of its ethos, structural organisation and operational practices follow from the premise that it is essentially a medical service. Care for people with all kinds of social and emotional problems is offered in what is unambiguously part of the medical system – in the UK, the National Health Service. Psychiatry and therefore the bulk of mental health services fall into the generic, medical basis on which physical health services are planned and delivered. This has the unfortunate consequence of meaning that social and psychological problems tend to be regarded as illnesses, even diseases. This means that a wide range of planning and commissioning decisions are made on this basis and, for the individual, medicalised solutions are the default response. So, people's problems tend to be classified into 'diagnoses' – despite the invalidity of that approach. Even psychologists' formulations tend to focus on what goes on inside rather than outside people's heads, concentrating on what individuals themselves are doing or not doing, and pathologising their responses rather than seeing their problems in a wider social context. In the current system, even when psychosocial interventions are offered, people are still given diagnoses such as 'conduct disorder' or 'post traumatic stress disorder'. Medication is offered routinely: as we've seen, the vast majority of people are offered medication and only medication.

From the top down, and from the bottom up, mental health care is currently predicated on a medical model. In the UK, the most influential single individual is the Medical Director of the National Commissioning Board. Mental healthcare is currently part of the medical infrastructure, which in the UK is the NHS. The Government's Department of Health provides funding and significant strategic direction, but more detailed decision-making is deferred to the 'arms-length' National Commissioning Board, the Medical Director of the Board, and the 25 National Clinical Directors. These expert clinical leaders provide expert advice and research on conditions and services, ranging from obesity and diabetes to emergency preparedness and critical care. This is all positive and necessary. But it does mean that mental healthcare falls under the directorship of a clinical director within this very medicalised structure and system. This 'clinical primacy' is also seen further down the system. NHS Trusts – the UK's core delivery units – have 'medical directors' to lead and guide services. While as individuals and as a group, medical directors – and the national clinical directors – perform a valuable service, any service run in and by a healthcare system will reflect the ethos and dominant methodologies of that system. This profoundly affects every aspect of our mental healthcare system. Indeed, even the term 'mental health care' conveys this medical dominance; psychological well-being may be a more appropriate phrase.

Immediately after I qualified as a clinical psychologist, I was asked by my boss to offer a psychological perspective to the construction of a new in-patient mental health unit. The hospital in which we worked was expanding and modernising, and a new in-patient unit was included in the plan. So I visited the manager responsible for commissioning the development and liaising with the architects. I hope that my perspective was useful (to be honest, the main thing that I suggested was to try to make sure that the unit was as dissimilar to a prison as possible). However, I was intrigued by the fact that the hospital manager was briefing the architects using an NHS document entitled something like 'guidance on the design of hospital wards'. It was, actually, quite helpful, but it also assumed that beds on hospital psychiatric wards naturally required all the paraphernalia of general hospital wards caring for people with serious physical health conditions. To the authors of this slim pamphlet, and therefore to my colleague, a ward was a ward was a ward, and a bed was a bed was a bed. In his carefully written brief for the architects, therefore, each bed was carefully supplied with an alarm button for the nurses, a vacuum (a nozzle allowing easy attachment of medical devices that require a vacuum), oxygen and other pipes and devices. I thought then, and I think now, that this is not the basis on which to plan psychological well-being services.

People with psychological problems of various kinds are not offered residential care lightly. People are likely to be acutely distressed, sometimes confused and often in despair. So we absolutely need to pay very careful attention to the design of their surroundings. It may be reasonable to have access to an emergency call button. It is obviously wise – as in any good hotel – to have plenty of power sockets. As I said earlier, we need to be careful about ligature points (places where someone who is contemplating suicide might be able to attach a means of ending their life). We would almost certainly want to ensure privacy but also that staff could achieve access to private places in an emergency. Planning for a residential unit for people in acute emotional distress will not be identical to planning a good hotel. But it clearly isn't the same as planning a conventional hospital ward. Things have improved over the 20 years that I have been qualified as a clinical psychologist, and more enlightened planning is now apparent. But it remains true that most in-patient psychiatric wards are planned, designed and operated as exactly that – as hospital wards for people who are ill. In a different system, predicated on different assumptions, residential units should be just as carefully planned, but planned on different assumptions, and the result would be very different.

In my experience, working as a clinical psychologist, this medical dominance has important consequences. Decision-making within organisations often reflects not only the external context, but also the specific and dominant role occupied by psychiatrists (individually often excellent, but nevertheless reflecting one particular perspective) in the hierarchy of the organisations. On a clinical level, key decisions are often made by consultant psychiatrists. Multi-disciplinary team meetings are often essentially only convened to discuss how those decisions should be implemented. In practice, those multi-disciplinary meetings are often strongly influenced by a biomedical perspective; it's instructive to observe what happens if the consultant psychiatrist is absent – frequently the meetings are postponed, or automatically led by a more junior psychiatrist.

But the care and support for people struggling with emotionally and psychologically challenging circumstances needs to be organised very differently. In place of this inappropriate medical service, we need a new, psychosocial one. There should be a network of community-based care teams, linked to social services provision and other local authority services, as well as to the NHS and third-sector organisations. Fortunately, that's the direction of travel nationally. There is a general intention to integrate mental health care, physical health care and social care. We've seen a major integration of GP services with wider community and social services, and – importantly – we've seen UK public health services transferred wholesale into local authority management. What I'm proposing takes those ideas and drives them forwards. Mental health and well-being should be a local authority-managed, social and community resource, not a medical and hospital-based service. So, psychiatry – the profession of psychiatry, psychiatrists and indeed all mental health services – needs to stop trying to 'diagnose' illnesses, and focussing on the social determinants of mental health. A social service with medical input, not a medical service with a bit of social work added on.

This does not mean dispensing with psychiatric colleagues nor denying their importance. In this model, psychiatrists' contribution would remain significant and important. But they would be consultants *to*, not in charge *of* those local teams. This echoes the principles of the 'New Ways of Working' project – itself initiated by psychiatry to address the needs of psychiatry. It also reflects the principles of Pat Bracken and colleagues' model of best practice for mental health care.[1] A good analogy here is the medical advisor to Manchester United Football Club. Proper medical care and advice is undoubtedly vital to such a physical, high-value organisation. It would be bizarrely risky for a multi-million pound, international business, based on the physical prowess of a small number of athletes, to ignore their physical health. Medical care is an essential element of any world-leading sporting body. But Sir Alex Ferguson (or his replacement, David Moyes, following Ferguson's retirement) would never have suggested that his medical consultant has authority over him in terms of management; she'll be a consultant *to* the team, not the manager *of* the team.

## The NHS

In the UK, just after the Second World War, there was a profound revolution in the provision of a wide range of social services. The National Health Service was founded in 1948 (established by an Act of Parliament passed in 1946, to explain a few anomalies with dates). The idea was controversial – many people (including doctors) were concerned about the idea of a nationalised, socialised system. Indeed, the British Medical Association formally opposed the idea of a national health service. But the general idea of a National Health Service had broad support – that, through a system of what is effectively general taxation, every citizen has immediate access to a comprehensive system of gold-standard healthcare free at the point of need. The details, however, were also a matter of debate. In particular, there were differences of opinion in respect to whether the network of healthcare providers should be organised through existing local authorities – that local authorities should manage their local hospitals and doctors under the auspices of the new proposed scheme – or through a new, national, structural organisation. For various reasons, it was eventually decided that the local authority solution was less attractive than the idea of a new, bespoke structure, and the NHS as we know it was born.

These complex discussions were largely (and understandably) driven by the needs of physical health services. But, of course, the management of mental health services followed. In a remarkably short period of time, the National Health Service (a structure independent of local authorities, city mayors and town Councils) was established. Even then, there was considerable discussion over whether mental health services should be part of this system. Some commentators took the view (a view I would now share) that mental health care and the physical health services brought under the new NHS were essentially different. They argued that mental health care should be separately organised and should fall under local authority control. There were three powerful arguments for inclusion of mental health care within the NHS. In conventional medical science and practice, psychiatry was (and it was argued had been for a long time) part of the profession of medicine. It was also argued – and this is an argument we've seen rehearsed many times – that conventional medical research was on the brink of revealing causal mechanisms and effective interventions that would enable much more effective, medical, treatment. And, more negatively, it was argued that local authorities were not sufficiently well-organised or well-resourced to meet the needs of people with mental health problems. So, mental health services in the UK were, and as we can see today still are, squarely located within the National Health Service.

That may well have been a necessary decision back in 1946 – when local authority administration was considerably different – but seems much less appropriate today. Since 1948, the network of community-based mental health services has experienced massive development. There is, now, a growing and positive relationship between on the one hand largely community-based NHS mental health trusts offering both traditional 'out-patient' services and residential 'in-patient' units and, on the other, the various social services provided by local authorities. The pattern of provision is highly complex. Healthcare is, rightly, an important part of our economy and an important element of our social provision, and there are many different specialist teams and services. So, for example – and this is definitely not an exhaustive list – the NHS offers specialist mental health care for new mothers (often delivered by community mental health trusts, but based in general hospitals or maternity hospitals) and child and adolescent mental health services (CAMHS), sometimes delivered by community mental health trusts, but occasionally by specialist children's hospitals. It offers a very wide range of services for people of working age – specialist learning difficulties services, services for people with physical disabilities, services for people with substance misuse problems, support for people returning to work, help for offenders who have mental health problems, and services for older people. There are even very specialist services for, for example, commercial sex workers, asylum seekers, war veterans and young people leaving local authority care. All these services interface with family doctors – GPs – and with similar, synergistic services offered by local authorities and third-sector organisations.

The close liaison between NHS and local authority services can be seen in what are called 'Section 75 arrangements'. For obvious and understandable reasons, local authorities and health services have developed (relatively) effective and efficient ways of working together. These are lubricated by Section 75 of the National Health Service Act (2006) – hence the name – which encourages health trusts and local authority social services departments to pool money, delegate functions to each other and to integrate their resources and management structures. This effectively means that a nurse, a psychologist or a psychiatrist could find themselves employed by an NHS Trust, but under day-to-day management by a local authority manager ... or vice-versa. This is seen as hugely advantageous to planning services across a wide range of areas of mental health care, but has so far been particularly used in learning disability services and in services for children and for older people.

This collaborative approach between health and local authority agencies is further strengthened by the development of local Health and Wellbeing Boards in the UK. In 2012 the UK Government introduced a highly controversial piece of legislation – the Health and Social Care Act 2012[2] – which was seen by many as a horrifying step towards privatisation of the NHS. But it also did something rather wonderful. It established, under statute law, Health and Wellbeing Boards in each major local authority. These Boards act as opportunities for NHS and local authority managers, as well as leaders and opinion-formers from the wider community to work together to improve the health and well-being of their local population and reduce health inequalities. These Health and Wellbeing Boards bring together clinical commissioning groups and local councils to develop a shared understanding of the health and well-being needs of the community – a Joint Strategic Needs Assessment (JSNA) – and a joint strategy for action. These Boards are designed to enable joint commissioning and integrated services across health and social care, joined-up services between the NHS and local councils, and stronger democratic legitimacy and engagement. Because local authorities are responsible for services such as housing and education, there is huge potential for fully-integrated services.

In my view, these initiatives are very positive and hopeful. Even as things stand, they offer great potential for improving mental health care. But things need to progress further down this route. Indeed, it offers what is effectively an escape route for psychiatry – a pathway away from crisis and contention towards a positive future. Mental health care should be a matter for local authorities. Psychiatry should be a proud and strong, valued and effective profession, offered as part of the services provided by local authorities for the benefit of their citizens.

## Public health and mental health

We have a good – proud and strong – example of this move in the UK. One key medical profession – public health – has recently transferred from health service management (back) into local authority control. I'm referring to public health working at the level of population and planning, rather than at the level of the individuals, to help a city or a community stay healthy, and to protect them from threats to their health. Public health professionals aim to improve health and quality of life through improving the way that we prevent and treat diseases. They aspire to the World Health Organization's aim: health as 'a state of complete physical, mental and social well-being and not merely the absence of disease or infirmity'. Public health, like mental health, is a team effort, with input from physicians, epidemiologists, statisticians, nurses, microbiologists, environmental health officers... even lawyers. Typical policies address things like reducing smoking and helping people to quit, reducing drugs misuse and dependence, giving all children a healthy start in life, reducing harmful drinking, planning for health emergencies such as epidemics and pandemics, screening for cancer, reducing obesity and improving diet, and promoting breastfeeding. Public health services, of course, also address mental health.

Until 2013, local public health services were organised from within the NHS – by Primary Care Trusts (PCTs). In a rather controversial move, the same legislation that introduced Health and Wellbeing Boards also transferred responsibility for public health services from the NHS (in this case PCTs) to local authority control. Although (at least in principle) the amount of taxpayers' funding available to public health was protected, and although the responsibilities for the public health service remain unchanged, public health services are now part of the infrastructure of local authorities.

This has, of course, been a challenging period for many of my colleagues in public health. In my view, however, local authority management is the right place for public health. Maybe an example will help explain why. Again it's from the city where I work, Liverpool. Part of Liverpool's civic pride includes the legacy of Dr William Duncan. Like most doctors in Victorian Britain, Duncan came from a privileged background. But, after qualifying as a doctor in 1829 and working as a GP or family doctor in a working class area of Liverpool, he became interested in the health of the poor and started researching the living conditions of his patients. He was shocked by the poverty he found, and in his observations of the clear link between housing conditions and the outbreak of diseases such as cholera, smallpox and typhus. Dr Duncan started a lifelong campaign for improved living conditions and, together with Liverpool's Borough Engineer, James Newlands, started to tackle the problems he saw. This led to his appointment as Liverpool's first Medical Officer of Health, and in the passing of Liverpool's Sanitary Act in 1846. Dr Duncan undertook all of this rather splendid activity without compromising his role as a doctor and this was an excellent use of his medical training, but it was all enacted through and with local civic authorities. So the recent move of public health services to local authority management is in keeping with the best traditions of the profession.

Public health professionals themselves stress the extent to which our health is socially determined. Many argue that by far the most effective policies are those enacted at the population level. Researchers point to the extent to which our health is a product of social factors, and particularly how social inequalities lead to inequalities in health outcomes. More importantly, perhaps, the most effective interventions are social interventions – health education and promotion campaigns to reduce smoking, alcohol use; improve unhealthy diets; improve take-up of immunisation; improve breast-feeding rates and condom use; reduce UV sunbed use to prevent melanoma; prohibit advertising of cigarettes and sales of alcoholic drinks aimed at young drinkers; promote campaigns on licensing laws, housing policies...some of the most important public health activities are central to local authority responsibilities. More importantly, interventions aimed at individuals are less effective, in many cases, than genuinely *public* health interventions. Three straightforward examples involve food, cigarettes and alcohol. It seems abundantly clear that nearly everyone in industrialised democracies understands the health risks associated with obesity, smoking and excessive drinking. But we all find it difficult to change our individual behaviour, and it is often difficult for health professionals to help us. Probably because most of us already understand the negative health consequences of our behaviour, it isn't very effective for health professionals merely to encourage us to eat less, to take more exercise or to stop smoking or drinking. We know that. The point is, however, that despite knowing it, we don't do it. Public health professionals believe that what is needed is more activity at the level of public bodies. We need to examine the way in which cities are constructed – encouraging public transport, cycling and walking. We need to look to taxation systems – to reward healthy eating and drinking and to put economic pressures on unhealthy choices. We need to look to regulation and licensing – addressing the advertising industries (especially where they target groups such as children) and food labelling (identifying hidden fats, salts and sugars in processed foods). And we need to look at local authority planning regulations and make choices about what and how we build, at least partly, on the basis of health considerations. The action of individuals is, of course, crucial. We all need to attend to our own health and the choices we can make as individuals. But the role of local authorities in public health is crucial.

The principal drivers for the changes in how UK public health services are organised and delivered, including the key move of public health from NHS to local authority management, are related to physical health. But the arguments for these changes are even more powerful in mental health. Even more than with physical health, there are strong social determinants of psychological well-being. Social, and particularly economic, inequalities are significant predictors of a wide range of problems. And the social and psychological mediators – including, but not limited to lifestyle factors – that accompany these social and economic inequalities are strong predictors of our psychological as much as our physical health. Many psychologists, psychiatrists and sociologists have pointed out how much of our mental health is dependent on the same social and economic pressures (and especially inequalities) as those which lead to problems with physical health. Perhaps more importantly, we know that crises such as divorce, marital difficulties, unemployment, stresses at work, financial difficulties, illnesses in family members, crime (both as a victim and as a perpetrator, when caught up in the criminal justice system), assaults, bullying and childhood abuse are all powerful direct causes of mental health problems. Street or recreational drug use is also often implicated, and it is abundantly clear that the abuse of street drugs is a quintessentially social problem. It is these factors, of course, that impel psychiatrists such as Pat Bracken and Phil Thomas to be such powerful advocates for 'social psychiatry'.

The same arguments apply to interventions. Nobody would deny the benefits of direct medical care. But progress in improving the health and well-being of citizens also requires intervention at the population level. In the case of physical health care, many of the most deadly killers – heart disease, diabetes, stroke, cancer, and sexually-acquired infections – need to be addressed through public health measures for maximum benefit. This is also true for mental health.

Therapy, even medication, may be helpful for some, but real improvements in the overall psychological health of the population require action at a societal level. We need to address the causes listed earlier. Because marital separation is a major source of emotional stress, we should be ensuring that there is sufficient support for people going through separation or marital difficulties: mediation services, support for single parents, and equitable laws concerning divorce proceedings and child custody. Because unemployment is a major source of distress, we should aim for full employment, and certainly do what we can to protect people from the emotional and economic impact of unemployment. Conversely, work-related stress is also a big issue for many people. We need to ensure equitable and supportive employment practices, including employee relations, a living wage, decent terms and conditions and appropriate employee representation. Services such as Citizens Advice (a Government-funded, but independent, network of advice agencies with offices in most towns across the UK), debt counselling agencies and Victim Support are vital to help people in financial difficulties, victims of crime and people dealing with a range of other traumatic life events. Similarly, drugs advice and drugs counselling services play vital roles in maintaining the well-being of citizens. Psychologists and psychiatrists throughout history have realised that our experiences in childhood are fundamentally important in determining future mental health problems, and that emotional neglect, bullying, and childhood emotional, physical and sexual abuse are all powerful direct causes of mental health problems. It is therefore vital that we, as a society, act to protect children – not merely mop up the emotional consequences later in life. This means developing coordinated services to support families and parents in difficulty. It means supporting teachers and educational psychologists in schools, and it means supporting a network of children's services. And, no matter how politically controversial it might be, we should press for social justice and in particular for a more equal society.

For all these reasons, I see local authorities as the right place for the management of psychological health care. I believe that mental health care will remain inappropriately dependent on a medical, disease-based, ethos so long as it is seen as another branch of medicine. I see the journey of public health from PCT management to local authority management as offering a pioneering route for the transfer of mental health care from hospital-based services to local authority control. This vision would see opportunities for GPs, properly trained in mental health care, to help support the well-being of their clients. It would obviously see many more clinical psychologists.... But, as with our medical colleagues, they would be working in the community, not in hospitals or 'clinics'. As mentioned earlier, medical psychiatrists would be consultants *to*, not in charge *of* those teams. I envisage psychology-led teams (with an appropriate mix of staff) delivering psychosocial services in the community, not psychiatrist-led teams with medical and nursing colleagues delivering medical services to the community.

Pregnancy is a suitable analogy here. Pregnant women (and their babies) often benefit from high-quality medical care, and both doctors (of various kinds) and midwives have vital roles to play. But pregnant women are not 'ill' by virtue of their pregnant status. Pregnancy is not an illness that should be diagnosed and treated. Pregnant women need the support and intervention of medical colleagues. Some more than others. When there are problems in pregnancy, the role of medical colleagues becomes greater. When pregnancies are unplanned and threaten a woman's well-being, again, the advice and assistance of medical colleagues is often vital. But we still do not regard a pregnant woman as 'ill' and we don't regard pregnancy as an 'illness'. Similar analogies can be made across the work of GPs as they deliver medical help to people in many facets of their lives. Similar analogies could be made with the work of medical colleagues as advisors to athletes. Medical science is invaluable as people fulfil their potential in all aspects of life. But an athlete does not have to be 'ill' to benefit from the advice of a team doctor.

## Support health and well-being, don't treat 'illness'

There is a purpose and a reason for arguing that mental health care, including psychiatry, should be located in the social services of local authorities. A mere change in the line of management would be pointless without a change in ethos and practice. The point of bringing mental health care under local authority control is to shift from a service based on a disease-model ethos to one based on a person-centred ethos: from one designed to treat mental illness to one designed to foster human well-being.

This isn't really too much to wish for. And it should also be close to the aspiration of psychiatrists. The 1948 founding Charter of the World Health Organization describes health as '…a state of complete physical, mental and social well-being and not merely the absence of disease or infirmity'. The European Commission takes a step further, describing mental health as: 'a resource which enables them to realise their intellectual and emotional potential, and to find and fulfil their roles in social, school and working life. For societies, good mental health of citizens contributes to prosperity, solidarity and social justice'. Interestingly, the European Commission also suggests that: 'the mental condition of people is determined by a multiplicity of factors including biological (e.g., genetics, gender), individual (e.g., personal experiences), family and social (e.g., social support) and economic and environmental (e.g., social status and living conditions)'.

The consequences of bullying and abuse in childhood can be far-reaching and lifelong. Children form their views about themselves and their futures during their adolescence, and all manner of negative life events can lead to significant future distress. The impact of childhood abuse – emotional abuse, neglect and both physical and sexual abuse – is huge. Children also spend a very significant amount of their time inter-acting with peers (with other children, usually in school or with school friends). Any observer of children will see how hierarchies and patterns of in-group and out-group behaviour are quickly established. These serve as frameworks within which children begin to understand their skills and talents, how others see them, and what patterns of friendship they can expect. These complex relationships are vital to their healthy emotional and psychological development...and bullying is therefore traumatic and has long-lasting consequences.

In our mental health services as they are currently constituted, these children tend to come to our attention when 'disorders' or 'illnesses' are diagnosed – whether as children or later as adults. Many colleagues working both in child and adolescent mental health services (CAMHS) and in adult psychiatric services stress the social determinants of later emotional problems, and most colleagues working in child psychiatry services are fully aware of the impact of social circumstances and trau-matic life events on children's emotional well-being. Similarly, many social psychiatrists are fully aware that emotional distress in adult life frequently stems from experiences in childhood. But nevertheless, and despite their close working relationships, the mental health system is currently somewhat separate from education and children's services and, crucially, based on different assumptions and ethos.

## Mental health care in an age of austerity

At the time of writing this book, a right-wing government in the UK has put all of public spending under huge strain. Central government financial support for local authorities has been substantially reduced, and social services are under considerable strain. Because of the great affection shown by UK citizens towards their health service – the NHS – government ministers have pledged to protect the funding for the health services (a pledge that, remarkably, seems not yet to have been broken). It seems to be a matter of pride to some in government that the UK is planning to reduce the funding for public services to a level not seen since 1948.[3] I must say that this is a matter of concern, if not shame, for me. All this means that local authorities are, as I write this, under unprecedented financial pressure. It is in this context of financial pressure that many of my colleagues have been concerned about the transfer of public health services to local authority control. The argument is that it is much better to keep such services within the ring-fenced NHS budget than to expose them to the pressures of a shrinking local authority funding model.

Whilst this is an important concern in the current UK context, it does not negate my wider argument. The temporary details of public service funding in the UK in 2014 should not prevent a larger debate about what the appropriate ethos and service model might be for mental health and well-being services more generally. In my opinion, any concern about the funding of and costs of services makes the case for integrated care even more strongly. To save unnecessary costs, we should do it right, first time, every time.

## Philosophies

The underpinning philosophy of traditional, 'disease-model' mental health care is, as my doctor colleague put it, that '...ultimately, our job is to treat illnesses'. Services suffer, and in my view often even do harm, because they start from that presumption. This is not helped by the frequent and insistent calls to see mental health in biological, reductionist terms. Such accounts ignore the links between the events in our lives, including in childhood, and our future mental health, suggesting instead that biological processes, pathologies and abnormalities are to blame. This stance was perhaps most acutely revealed in the suggestion made by the person I mentioned earlier who had been asked to review a paper submitted by colleagues of mine exploring the links between childhood sexual abuse and future psychotic experiences. They suggested that the apparent link could actually be a result of the children having a genetic abnormality that not only increased their risk of future psychosis but also actually made them more vulnerable to abuse! This contorted logic serves to minimise the link between childhood trauma and future mental health problems. It serves to exonerate abusers. It minimises the effects of abuse and denies society's responsibility to its victims. And it leaves our efforts to protect children disconnected from our attempts to help those who are suffering the after-effects of abuse either as children or in their later adult lives. Of course not all psychiatrists think like this, especially the colleagues behind what I am terming the 'Bracken Manifesto'. But this way of thinking does endure.

One of its effects is that access to services – as children or adults – is at least partially dependent on meeting diagnostic criteria for a 'disorder' – in other words, being seen as 'mentally ill' in some way. This is especially the case in those countries where insurance companies fund help for people: they will often only do so on the basis of a 'diagnosis'. However, even in the UK access to services is increasingly dependent on such labels. This offends against basic psychological and psychiatric science – we know that events in our childhood and social life affect our emotions and mental health, and it is inappropriate to separate the two. It is also profoundly unhelpful, leaving both children and adults not only dealing with stigmatising labels that suggest that they are defective in some way, but in the invidious position of either accepting these labels or missing out on care. And, vitally, it distracts us from the urgent need for preventative action.

It is unacceptable to see that children are being abused and bullied, and then to wait before offering psychological help until the evidence of harm is sufficient to meet the criteria for a 'mental disorder'. I do not believe that this is what anybody wants. I do not even think that this is in the minds of those misguided individuals who minimise the links between trauma and subsequent mental health problems. And yet this is the consequence of three unfortunate factors: firstly a mental health care system still dominated by a biomedical reductionist ethos and a 'disease-model' mentality, secondly a consequent 'diagnose–treat' approach in which access to services is based upon meeting the criteria for a so-called 'mental illness', and thirdly a separation of mental health services from other social services.

## Radical measures

We can either see mental health problems as essentially medical conditions with social elements, or as essentially social problems with medical aspects. Of course medical, biological factors play a role. But I believe it is right to see mental health difficulties as essentially social problems.

Care for people with emotional and psychological problems should therefore be part of the social service offered by local authorities. The present multi-disciplinary teams managed by healthcare trusts (and similar hospital-based services in countries other than the UK) should be transferred to local authority control. This transfer could happen in a dramatic fashion – with central government legislation mandating a wholesale transfer of assets and responsibilities. Alternatively, it could happen more gradually – with local authorities tendering, and being awarded contracts, for the delivery of mental health care. In the UK, with increased commercialisation of our National Health Service, this could be a very real possibility. This would retain the services of medical, psychiatric colleagues, but world employ them differently. We would expect an over-arching ethos based on promoting well-being rather than treating illness, and a greater focus on the social determinants of mental health. There would be a greater focus on psychosocial interventions, although, of course, these teams would need to have plentiful, varied, high-quality treatment options. It is clear, however, that this would profoundly change our relationship with traditional psychiatry.

This proposal is radical, and will be opposed by many psychiatrists. It is relatively well known that at the point when the NHS was founded, there was considerable debate over whether mental health services should be included. Most psychiatrists passionately believe that it would have been a disaster if mental health had not been included with the bulk of mainstream, physical health – medicine. This is a genuine and honourable belief. And it is possible that, back in 1948, local authority structures would not have been robust enough to provide the services that vulnerable people need. But what might have been right in 1948 is not necessarily right now. And it is possible that some of the passion with which psychiatrists argue that mental health must remain wedded to physical health may have more to do with their profession than their patients. Nick Craddock and colleagues, in their manifesto for old-fashioned, biomedical, psychiatry, demon-strated this point clearly. For at least some psychiatrists, remaining part of a very medical community appears central to their professional identity and to their confidence that their role will remain protected. So I imagine that very many psychiatrists will be highly alarmed at the suggestion that they, their profession, and the services in which they work should be transferred out of the 'medical' community and into the 'social care' community.

I suspect that many people in the pharmaceutical and insurance industries (at least outside of the EU, in nations where insurance-based rather than state-provided healthcare is more common) would be equally concerned. The global pharmaceutical industry makes enor-mous profit from the sale of drugs to healthcare organisations – and to patients themselves – and healthcare insurers similarly profit from the commercial aspects of a system that treats emotional problems as if they were 'illnesses like any other'. It is obvious that ideas such as those I am suggesting here would threaten that approach. I am directly challenging the notion that mental health problems can be treated as if they were similar physical illnesses; I am suggesting that a medical approach to care is inappropriate; I am arguing for a significantly reduced reliance on medication; and I am suggesting that the healthcare industry is not the right location for services. If implemented, this would be a major impact on the profit-base of important and influential commercial companies. Nevertheless, that is what I believe is right.

Unfortunately, all that means there may be trouble. The medical and psychiatric communities are powerful – with well-established and effective professional bodies, and statutory mechanisms for catching and holding the ears of policymakers. But, despite the likely opposition, this aspect of my prescription will remain – to move mental health care from medical to social management, from the health service to local authority control.

# 8
## Can We Afford It?

*Adoption of a psychosocial model, and implementation of the reforms recommended here, would result in much lower reliance on medical interventions, and a much greater reliance on social and psychological interventions. The net cost of such changes is likely to be minimal and could offer opportunities for greater investment in care and support for some of the most vulnerable in society.*

In a just world, this chapter would be redundant. The UK is a wealthy nation – the world's sixth-largest economy (or perhaps eighth-largest when you take international financial exchange rates into account). It has a moral duty to spend some of that wealth on the general benefit of its citizens, especially in times of economic difficulty. As I mentioned in the introductory chapter, the World Health Organization now regards mental health problems as the leading cause of disability worldwide, and has estimated that they cost as much as $2,500 billion worldwide in 2010. In the UK, around 6,000 people take their own lives each year, and mental health issues have been estimated as costing the UK economy as much as £105 billion each year. So it's worth spending some money on truly effective services.

I do in fact think we should spend more on mental health care – I believe we should spend more on health and social care generally.[1] The United Kingdom spends about £100 billion per year on healthcare, or about £2,000 per person per year.[2] Of that, around 14% goes on mental health. It's worth pointing out that the UK's NHS is one of the world's least expensive healthcare systems, despite being universal and free at the point of need. It's equally worth pointing out that comparable costs of healthcare in the USA are twice as high, and yet a third of US citizens experience financial barriers to affordable healthcare such as out-of-pocket charges and high insurance premiums.³ So investment in healthcare generally, and in mental health and well-being more particularly would not be unreasonable.

Moreover, many would argue that investment in such services would be cost-effective. The IAPT programme (discussed in Chapter 4) was powerfully supported by Lord Richard Layard, a well-connected Labour peer and leading academic economist, on the grounds that investment in psychological therapies would be cost-effective. Similarly, it has been suggested that evidence-based parenting support for families could prevent mental health problems in later life and therefore save money, and that a programme of work specifically focussing on helping parents deal with child behaviour problems has been estimated to cost £210 million but save £5.2 billion. Most interestingly, economists have suggested that care delivered outside of 'mental health services' could be particularly promising; it has been estimated that better mental health support in the workplace could save UK businesses up to £8 billion a year.⁴

## Costs and savings

Arguments about the overall health budgets, and about the relative proportion of that spending on mental health and well-being are political decisions. In my judgement, the UK's National Health Service, free at the point of use, universal and comprehensive, providing gold-standard healthcare for all and funded from general taxation is an example of enlightened and human civilisation that deserves nothing short of protection, support and replication worldwide. I believe that we in the UK would be well advised to spend slightly more on healthcare (given that our costs as a proportion of overall government spending are slightly below average for developed nations). In particular, I believe that it would be worth investing more in mental health and well-being services. Because people play an important role in their own health – through the type of lifestyle they lead – such investment would be of net benefit to the nation, reducing future health and social care costs.

But the reforms that my colleagues and I are advocating do not depend on extra funding. Indeed, they may even save money. Importantly, we need to make different spending decisions. We are certainly recommending change, but the changes we recommend need not be expensive.

In a nutshell, we would like to see society beginning to acknowledge that so-called 'mental health problems' are essentially psychological and social, and providing psychological and social services to improve psychological (and physical) well-being. To that end, we need to see a network of professionals skilled in psychosocial interventions and coordinated by Health and Well-being Boards within local authorities. There should be close liaison between those professionals and our medical colleagues in primary care. The majority of these proposals are cost-neutral: a shift from hospital in-patient wards to residential units commissioned by local authorities and based on a social model may not save huge sums, but neither is it likely to be hugely expensive. A wholesale transfer of mental health care from NHS trusts to local authorities' social care services would have some costs in the transition itself but the baseline costs would not rise. Implementing this plan would result in much lower reliance on medical interventions, and a much greater reliance on social and psychological interventions. In this vision, to be precisely clear, we would need fewer psychiatrists. We would need fewer medical professionals assuming leadership of clinical teams, because the ethos would no longer be predominantly medical. And although we would certainly want better physical health care, we would look to our primary care (GP) colleagues for much of that consultation, linking psychological care to people's wider well-being. We would, in contrast, require much greater emphasis on, training in, and staffing of, psychosocial approaches.

In summary, I am recommending: a transfer of mental health services to local authorities (including a shift from hospital to residential care), substantial reduction in the prescription of medication, a shift of medical responsibility from psychiatry to GPs with commensurate reduction in psychiatrist numbers, the training or retraining in a more psychosocial approach of a large number of current mental health workers and, perhaps, the recruitment of a number of additional clinical psychologists. For the avoidance of doubt, I would welcome more investment both in social services and in psychosocial aspects of mental health and well-being, but my proposals for the reform of care systems do not merely involve throwing money at the problem, rather more a refocussing of resources, and instead are sensible and eminently affordable.

## The excitingly named 'transitional support funds'

If we were to shift responsibility for mental health and well-being services to their most appropriate place – local authorities – then there would be some costs involved. We can estimate these costs, described by civil servants as 'transitional support funds', by looking at the recent transfer, in the UK, of public health units from health services management into local authorities (as described in Chapter 7). Health and social care systems differ very considerably from nation to nation. That makes it slightly difficult to translate costs of service change from one jurisdiction to another. However, it is useful to know that the UK Secretary of State for Health allocated a sum of £15m to fund the transition of public health services.[5] This sum was not, of course, intended to fund the services themselves, but to cover all the necessary costs involved in the physical transfer of services (legal costs, planning costs, the physical costs of moving, employment costs, office rental etc.). This is a surprisingly small sum, but does appear to have been sufficient for a relatively efficient transfer of responsibilities. It could be argued that mental health services are a much larger, much more complex, proposition than public health services – they employ many more people, in many more settings, doing very different tasks, including life-saving clinical services. So any transitional costs are likely to be much greater than the sums involved in public health. To be conservative, therefore, it might be reasonable to assume that the one-off costs involved in the transfer of legal responsibilities, employment and management systems, and so on, could be as high as £100m. These would, again, be one-off costs, and £100m is around 0.8% of the annual budget for mental health care in the UK. Other costs of the reforms I am proposing would, however, be recurrent.

## Greater investment in psychology, social workers, therapists

Central to my proposal is the recommendation that we significantly increase the number of people skilled in psychosocial interventions and, vitally, psychosocial approaches to mental health and well-being. This is very much the province of the IAPT – Improving Access to Psychological Therapies – programme that I discussed in Chapter 4. I discussed, earlier, how my proposals differ from the IAPT programme in significant ways. But some lessons can be learned from their health economic arguments. I agree with Lord Richard Layard that a reasonable target for the UK should be to increase the number of people capable of offering psychological and psychosocial help by an extra 10,000.[6] However, in the vision I am offering here, I would not expect all 10,000 to be new employees of the health and social care system. Many would be people who had worked in the old system and then re-trained in the approach outlined here. We need to separate the costs of employing new, additional, staff from the costs of re-training existing staff.

Although we need more people qualified and available to deliver the range and scope of evidence-based psychosocial interventions discussed in the previous chapter, this does not mean simply employing many more people in addition to the existing staff (which would be very expensive indeed) or laying-off large numbers of people in order to change the staffing profile. In our vision, we would take a large current workforce of medical and nursing colleagues, and transform them to a large, effective, humane workforce working in genuinely multidisciplinary teams. This should happen in the context of a major change in ethos. We are not only proposing transferring people from NHS employment to local authority employment (from governance by the CCGs, the clinical commissioning groups, to HWBs, health and well-being boards, in arcane UK governance speak) but also explicitly re-orienting their work and retraining. The current focus on medical ideology, the 'disease model', diagnosis, and medical treatment is part of the problem. In the current, 'disease-model' framework, it seems to make sense to spend a very great deal of money on people employed to deliver medical care. But we are suggesting something very different. Instead of 'nursing' or 'medical' staff, we would see a great deal of the day-to-day care delivered by staff trained primarily in psychological and social care. That would mean re-training existing staff (particularly nurses) as CBT therapists, social pedagogues, and (properly trained, properly supervised) experts in the wider range of interventions discussed earlier. We would like to see residential centres ('in-patient units') being places of safety and calm; drawing much less on the tradition of medical wards. In particular, any reduced reliance on coercion in mental health is likely to result in significant cost savings – it is very expensive to provide coercive care, with the heavy reliance on high staffing levels and physical security. But in the vision of care we are proposing here, medical doctors would still be available for consultation about prescribing, as would pharmacist colleagues – whom I've always regarded as crucial members of any team that involves prescribing decisions; pharmacists are (excuse the pun) indispensible!

That would take some training resource, but it wouldn't mean more staff. It is clear that there are opportunities for leadership by clinical psychologists in these proposals. But the proposal is not in fact that everybody should have one-to-one psychotherapy from a large new cohort of clinical psychologists. We are, at most, suggesting that psychologists help to coordinate care – with social workers as well as clinical psychologists taking a very clear lead on these issues. We are not suggesting that we need clinical psychologists to deliver every aspect of the social and psychological care described earlier. Many of my colleagues would like to see clinical psychologists leading these changes – offering clinical leadership in community teams, developing multi-factorial, multi-agency formulations, and in leading, training and supervising CBT therapists. This would apply, of course, in residential units, where again our skills in formulation should come to the fore. This, in my opinion, would also apply to care offered under a Mental Health Act (so long as this was predicated, as I have argued earlier, on the principles of autonomy, decision-making capacity and legal oversight) and where clinical psychologists and nurses already have the responsibility to coordinate care.

Nevertheless, there are training costs, and it would be remiss to ignore the benefits of greater investment in properly qualified staff.

## Training and re-training

To execute this vision, we will need to see significant investment in the training of psychosocial approaches and clinical leadership, especially in GPs and nursing colleagues. In the UK, mental health nursing is the largest profession by numbers, with around 48,000 mental health nurses (around 18,000 working in community settings and a massive 30,000 working in in-patient care). They are supported by about 55,000 support staff (4,500 in community settings and 50,500 in in-patient settings). As a comparison, by the way, there are around 8,000 clinical psychologists with 3,500 support staff.

It remains official Department of Health policy that our nursing colleagues 'should incorporate the broad principles of the Recovery Approach into every aspect of their practice' and 'use their valuable skills in the most effective way possible'.[7] This seems easy to translate into investment in training in evidence-based psychological and social therapies. In essence, the vision of care proposed here would see mental health nursing transformed from an adjunct to medical practice to a vehicle through which psychosocial interventions are delivered. All this supports the idea that we actually do have sufficient staff, just (in our view) doing many of the wrong things.[8] Our vision would lead to a very significant change in people's actual practice. So the question then is: how much would it cost to retrain them?

This is a very difficult question to answer precisely. The training of nurses, doctors – clinical psychologists too – is complex and the 'mental health' elements are not always easy to separate from more generic training. But in very general terms, the UK system for funding education and training is coordinated by an arms-length body of the Department of Health, 'Health Education England' (with parallel arrangements in the other nations).[9] The total annual budget for Health Education England is £4.9 billion. This pays for all training in healthcare, including medical education and that of nearly all undergraduate and postgraduate healthcare professions (although not the initial psychology degrees of clinical psychologists). It also pays for the post-qualification training of these professions.

That leaves us in the difficult position of estimating how much it would cost to commission a very significant retraining programme in mental health. We might suggest that mental health absorbs perhaps 10% of the total budget (in line with clinical spending ratios), so perhaps around £500 million a year. Many people might argue that the changes needed would be so radical that all training would need to change. Even then, that would not necessarily mean more training, just different training. The training of new professionals should encompass new material, new ideas, but would not necessarily be more expensive. However, there would be a short-term extra cost: that of retraining existing staff. A reasonable estimate might be that this would absorb up to an extra 20% of the notional 'mental health' training and education budget. That would mean our proposals could add up to £100 million to the bill.

Thus far, then, we could be looking at maybe a one-off £100 million for 'transitional support funds' and recurrent costs of maybe £100 million per annum for training.

## New staff?

So how many of the proposed '10,000 extra therapists' should be new staff? Our argument is that the system of care should be reformed, not that a new, parallel, system be developed in addition. So we may not need to assume that a vast new army of psychologists and clinical psychologists needs to be recruited. However, to ensure that proper care is, indeed, available, new staff would be welcome.

Any assumptions here will be crude, but using standard NHS pay scales[10] we could assume that an extra 1,000 clinical and other applied psychologists could cost an additional £70 million per year, and it would cost slightly less (perhaps £30 million) to employ an extra 1,000 psychological and other therapists in more junior roles. That might bring our notional costs for revolutionary change in mental health care to perhaps £200 million per year in addition to the notional £100 million transitional costs. But it is important to repeat that many health economists argue that investment in psychological therapies pays for itself.[11]

## Proper GP provision, proper physical healthcare

A key part of our vision for better care includes the provision for real physical health care. Bizarrely, despite the fact that psychiatrists' role as medical professionals, and consequently their potential to address physical health care needs, is frequently advanced as a reason for their 'clinical primacy' in teams, the physical health of mental health service users is frequently very poor. As we discussed above, therefore, a preferable model might be to look to our GP (primary care) colleagues to deliver this care – and indeed much of the medical aspects of what is currently the province of psychiatry.

That argument was made in Chapter 7, but it is reasonable here to consider the costs of such a change. There are three principal ways to consider this. It could be argued that such care is, or should be, part of the GPs' responsibilities. But we need to consider the resource implications. It could be argued that as GP colleagues adopt this responsibility, resources currently used to employ and support specialist psychiatrists could be redirected to employ and support additional primary care specialists – perhaps specialised, particularly, in mental health and well-being. In essence, this would imply a like-for-like redistribution of costs between primary care and psychiatry, with no net costs. In this sense, our proposals are (again) cost neutral. But it also seems reasonable to estimate the level of resources needed, not least to estimate the challenges involved. It is relatively simple (if hugely contentious) to suggest a like-for-like reduction in psychiatrist numbers and an increase in GP numbers, but what sort of numbers would be involved?

One possible comparison is to look at the costs of providing out-of-hours primary care cover. In the UK (which admittedly may be somewhat unrepresentative) we offer a comprehensive primary care service (delivered by the general practitioners or GPs that are repeatedly mentioned). Many years ago, these medical practitioners were tacitly expected to deliver a service 24 hours a day. More recently (and amid some controversy), plans were laid to establish out-of-hours services. Physical health care for people receiving mental health and well-being services could never be designed on exactly the same basis as out-of-hours GP services, but the scale of resources involved could give an indication of what might be required. Helpfully, this has already been estimated. The UK Department of Health estimates[12] that GP out-of-hours services cost around £500 million per year.

Not all of this sum is made up of salary costs, but it allows us a reasonable estimate as to what it might cost to implement our vision for transformed mental health services in the real world. If it costs about £500 million per year to provide out-of-hours primary care cover, it is reasonable to assume that a similar sum would be more than sufficient to meet the needs of people in receipt of mental health and well-being services. But extra expenditure is not really the point. Our vision involves a much clearer location of many of the medical responsibilities associated with mental health care within primary care. This is an argument for redistribution of resources, not extra resources. Since the salary costs of GPs, medical practitioners specialist in primary care, and psychiatrists, medical practitioners specialist in a different branch of medicine, will be fundamentally identical, this resource should be seen not as a net extra cost, but as a redistribution of funds. There are currently around 41,000 GPs working in the UK,[13] who would of course also be recipients of extra training. An increase of some 5,000 would therefore represent an increase of some 12%. That is reassuring, as it (again) is close to the overall proportion of healthcare spend dedicated to mental health issues.

Thus far then, in this economic argument, we might expect one-off 'transitional support costs' of £100 million, extra training costs of £100 million per annum to permit the re-deployment of nursing and medical staff to support psychosocial approaches, the cost of 2,000 entirely new staff specialising in psychological and psychosocial approaches at perhaps £100 million per annum, and perhaps £500 million per annum to provide for additional primary care cover, with this latter figure recouped partially from the existing spend on psychiatry, and partially from other sources.

## Less 'disease model', fewer psychiatrists

One of my psychiatric colleagues has called for the '...total dissolution of psychiatry...' and argued (as I mentioned in Chapter 6) that '...in an ideal world, I don't think [psychiatry] would exist...' While that might be an extreme position, the vision of care offered here proposes a comprehensive shift from a 'disease model' of care to a psychosocial model. That does indeed mean a redistribution of resources from medical to psychosocial provision. A substantial rebalancing of staffing resources along these lines would mean increased GP provision at the cost of a net reduction in psychiatrist numbers, and a substantial net reduction in the use of psychiatric medication. It is important, then, to see how such a redistribution of resources might impact on psychiatry.

In our analysis of a reconfigured service, proportionate cost savings would imply a net reduction of – importantly – both doctors and support staff from psychiatry to primary care. This means, psychiatrists, nursing support colleagues, and other support staff. There are currently some about 7,711 psychiatrist posts in the UK (according to an estimate in 2011[14]) of which 4,394 are at consultant level. This means that there is a ratio of about six nurses and seven support staff members for each psychiatrist. We have already seen that a transfer of a considerable proportion of medical care from 'psychiatry' to specialist primary care physicians with an interest in mental health could cost perhaps £500 million a year. If we were to resource such a sum entirely from staffing changes (which of course in the real world would be unreasonably harsh), some very basic assumptions about salary costs would imply that such a change would equate to the reinvestment of the resources associated with 1,000 psychiatrists and their associated support staff.

Some colleagues would press for greater, more radical, change. So some might argue for much more of the resource currently invested in around 7,700 psychiatrists to be transferred elsewhere. In the vision for mental health care and well-being that we are proposing, the change in ethos (from a 'disease model' to a psychosocial model) and the transfer of responsibilities from the medical services to local authority social services would strongly support a wholesale shift in staffing and activity.

But change is painful. While we might wish for transformational change, we need to be realistic. And even with relatively modest changes, there are significant training needs. So we should walk before we try to run. Is a shift of the resources associated with perhaps 1,000 psychiatrists in the UK achievable? Well, simply, yes!

Our best estimates suggest that there are perhaps 242 unfilled psychiatrist posts in the UK, 124 of them at consultant level. In addition, at least in 2010, there were also 420 posts filled by locums.[15] Locum psychiatrists are (hugely expensive) temporary staff contracted to offer cover, for unfilled posts. Using the figures above, a moratorium on these 662 posts would yield resources equivalent to around £331 million pounds a year. And that's just a moratorium on vacant posts. Of course, these opportunities for reinvestment are not simply cash sums generated by laying-off a certain number of psychiatrists and employing an equivalent number of GPs. Instead, we must be thinking about planning for an entire service re-design as outlined both here and in earlier chapters. The point, however, is that relatively modest changes in staffing profiles could easily sustain the £500 million resource demanded by the provision of a great deal of medical care by GP or primary care colleagues.

Since the problems we are discussing are not primarily medical in nature, the diagnoses are invalid and the drugs often don't work...we could easily afford a different model of care if we make some difficult, but obvious, decisions.

At the risk of sounding repetitive, our economic argument now includes one-off 'transitional support costs' of £100 million, additional costs of £100 million per annum for extra training in psychosocial approaches, and perhaps £100 million per annum to meet the cost of 2,000 entirely new staff. The £500 million per annum cost of much greater reliance on primary care colleagues to offer physical health care, as well as clinical input as specialist medical practitioners, would be met by proportionate savings elsewhere in the staffing budget, predominantly traditional psychiatry. Critics (who would, presumably, object to many of these proposals) would point out that we would still see a net cost of some £200 million per annum. But rationalisation – and redeployment – of staffing resources are not the only possible routes to supporting the proposals outlined here.

## Less medication, fewer prescriptions

We saw in Chapter 3 that a rational and humane approach to mental health and well-being should involve a much more cautions, more pragmatic, more expert but more restrained, limited and short-term use of psychotropic medication. This, unequivocally, would involve a net reduction in the use of these very expensive drugs. So, what impact could this have on budgets?

As we also saw in Chapter 3, we spend around £800 million per year in the UK on prescriptions for psychotropic, psychiatric drugs. So a 25% shift in prescribing practices might yield £200m in net savings. Of course, all reduction in prescriptions would yield proportionate savings in costs. Given the ineffectiveness of medical treatments for social problems, it seems reasonably safe to conclude that (unlike investment in other forms of services) these savings will not lead to extra expenses elsewhere. I should be clear: in an ideal world I would like to see a very significant reduction in the use of such medication. In a realistic, but attractive, world, that could easily be reflected in a 50% saving – or £400 million per year.

In other words, our proposals would save money – would liberate resources for greater investment in mental health and well-being.

# 9
# A Manifesto for the Reform of Mental Health and Well-being Services

*The need for reform in mental health services is acute, severe and unavoidable. This demands nothing less than a manifesto for reform.*

A spectre is haunting our mental health services. Recent scientific advances in understanding human psychology have revealed traditional 'disease-model' thinking about mental health to be profoundly flawed, and far-reaching changes are required in how we plan and commission services. Our present approach to helping people in acute emotional distress is severely hampered by old-fashioned and unscientific ideas about the nature and origins of mental health problems, and vulnerable people suffer as a result of inappropriate treatment. Radical remedies are required.

Taking its lead from physical health care, the current mental health care system currently 'diagnoses' our emotional, behavioural and psychological problems as 'illnesses', and is largely based on the idea that they arise primarily from brain abnormalities. The hope has been that eventually 'biomarkers' (physical signs) and biological causes (preferably genetic) will soon be found. This 'disease model' underpins too much of modern mental health care and has had profound and damaging effects.

It has led to inappropriate and harmful treatment. For many people, the only or main treatment currently offered is medication. Whilst useful for some people, recent research suggests that in general, the helpfulness of medication has been overestimated. Evidence is also accumulating that psychiatric medication can have dangerous adverse effects (side-effects) especially when taken long term.

It has prevented effective help and treatment. The disempowering idea that they are passive recipients of medical treatment for a disease has interfered with people's ability to help and support themselves and each other. It has diverted resources away from effective sources of help such as listening and psychological therapy services, and practical help to improve life circumstances.

It has led to alienation between staff and service users. When people are experiencing huge distress and fear that their sanity, even their life, is threatened, empathy and compassion are central to any attempt to help. The 'disease model' locates problems within the individual and leads staff to see people's behaviour and distress as irrational rather than as potentially understandable. This reduces professionals' ability to listen, empathise and show compassion. Service users' experiences are disregarded and their stories unheard. People often experience services as inhumane and avoid them. Only in mental health is there a 'survivor movement' – survivors not only of distress but specifically of the services supposedly established to help them.

It has necessitated widespread use of coercion. Mental health law has traditionally been based on the disease idea. Service users who see their problems differently and do not wish to take drugs have been seen as 'lacking insight' and have often been detained and administered drugs by force. Many thousands of people each year are detained in hospital and treated against their will. There is good reason to believe that these numbers could be reduced hugely if services adopted the approach outlined below.

It has diverted resources from efforts at prevention. The current approach to mental health care focusses attention almost exclusively on individual 'pathology' as the source of problems and as the focus for professional efforts. New knowledge about the role of life circumstances will lead to much more effective programmes of prevention, comparable to the effects on physical health of public health interventions such as the purification of drinking water.

The time has come for a wholesale reform of mental health services. We must move away from the 'disease model', which assumes that emotional distress is merely symptomatic of biological illness, and instead embrace a model of mental health and well-being that recognises our essential and shared humanity.

## The manifesto

### Article 1: services should be based on the premise that the origins of distress are largely social

The first step towards a humane, scientific approach to care is to change the framework of understanding from a 'disease model' to a 'psychosocial

model'. The guiding idea underpinning mental health services needs
to change from assuming that our role is to treat 'disease' to appreci-
ating that our role is to help and support people who are distressed as a
result of their life circumstances, and how they have made sense of and
reacted to them.

We all differ in the ways we respond to events, and there are many
reasons for those differences. Our thoughts, our emotions, our behaviour,
and therefore our mental health, are largely dependent on our understanding of the world, our thoughts about ourselves, other people, the
future and the world. There are as many different reasons for these different
responses as there are people in the world. Biological factors, social factors,
circumstantial factors – our learning as human beings – all affect us; those
external factors impact on the key psychological processes that help us
build up our sense of who we are and the way the world works.

### Article 2: services should replace 'diagnoses' with straightforward descriptions of problems

We must stop regarding people's very real emotional distress as merely
the symptom of diagnosable 'illnesses'. A simple list of people's problems (properly defined) would have greater scientific validity and would
be more than sufficient as a basis for individual care planning and for
the design and planning of services. Some medical professionals and
many members of the general public mistakenly believe that psychiatric
diagnoses reflect real 'illnesses'. However, research does not support this
view. There is little evidence that mental health 'diagnoses' say anything
useful about the causes of a problem or what is likely to help. Some
people have found 'diagnoses' useful in providing a framework within
which to understand their difficulties, and in accessing help and support.
However, there are other, more scientifically valid and more helpful ways
of reassuring people that their problems are recognised (in both senses
of the word), understood, validated, explained (and explicable) and that
some help is available. The approach described here outlines how this
vital help and support can continue to be provided without the need to
make the assumption that problems reflect underlying 'illnesses'.

Some legal and other professionals mistakenly believe that diagnoses
are needed in order to allow people to communicate efficiently with
one another. However again diagnoses are misleading and unnecessary;
a simple and direct list of a person's actual experiences and problems
provides more information and is of greater communicative value than
a diagnostic label. Of course we need to research the nature, causes and
remedies of problems. Again, 'diagnoses' are misleading here: rather

than trying to investigate hypothetical 'illnesses', researchers would be better advised to study the nature and causes of specific, identified problems, and what can help.

Many medical professionals and policymakers mistakenly assume that we need to use diagnoses in order to allocate resources to those who need them. However we can see from how resources are successfully allocated in a vast swathe of other public services that this simply isn't true.

### Article 3: services should radically reduce use of medication, and use it pragmatically rather than presenting it as 'treatment'

We should sharply reduce our reliance on medication to address emotional distress. Medication should be used sparingly and on the basis of what is needed in a particular situation – for example to help someone to sleep or to feel calmer. We should not look to medication to 'cure' or even 'manage' non-existent underlying 'illnesses'.

In practical terms, we should aim for a massive reduction in the level of psychiatric prescription. There should be many fewer prescriptions, at lower doses, for much shorter periods. In essence, this means adopting a 'drug-based' approach in contrast to the more common 'disease-based' approach. We should respond to people's specific symptoms, rather than make the mistake that we're treating illnesses that can be identified by diagnosis. We need to listen to the person's own experiences of which drugs have helped in the past and how they are finding those currently prescribed, and use what they say to guide our prescribing. Perhaps most importantly, we should only use psychiatric medication in the very short term (i.e., for a matter of days) in the vast majority of cases.

### Article 4: services should tailor help to each person's unique and complex needs

Problems do not come in neat boxes. Services should be equipped to help with the full range of people's social, personal and psychological needs, and to address both prevention and recovery.

We must offer services that help people to help themselves and each other rather than disempowering them: services that facilitate personal 'agency' in psychological jargon. That means involving a wide range of community workers and psychologists in multidisciplinary teams, and promoting psychosocial rather than medical solutions. Where individual therapy is needed, effective, formulation-based (and therefore individually tailored) psychological therapies should be available to all.

All such therapies should be evidence-based and delivered by qualified, competent professionals. Decisions about what therapy or therapies should be offered to whom should be based on a person's specific problems and on the best evidence for the effectiveness of the intervention, not on the diagnosis. Individual formulations should be used to put together an individualised package of care for each person's unique set of problems. Using psychological therapies as part of a psychosocial, rather than biomedical, approach would significantly change the way clinical psychologists and others work.

Our psychiatric colleagues would play an important medical role within this overall psychosocial ethos. Their role would be analogous to those of general practitioners, public health physicians, and doctors who offer their expertise to athletes.

### Article 5: services should offer care rather than coercion

When people are in crisis, residential care may be needed, but this should not be seen as a medical issue. Since a 'disease model' is inappropriate, it is also inappropriate to care for people in hospital wards; a different model of care is needed. As with other services, residential units should be based on a psychosocial rather than a medical model. Residential social workers or nurses who have retrained in a psychosocial approach (and possibly with a more appropriate professional title) are likely to be best placed to lead such units. The nature of extreme distress means medical colleagues may well be valuable members of the team but again their role should be as consultants *to* the team, rather than automatically as leaders *of* the team.

The need for compulsory detention would be much reduced within this new approach. In those instances where compulsory detention was necessary, decisions would be based on the risks that individuals are thought to pose to themselves and others, together with their capacity to make decisions about their own care. This approach is already the basis for the law in Scotland. The law in England and Wales permits the 'responsible clinician' (the person who is legally responsible for someone's care, traditionally a psychiatrist) to be a psychologist, nurse, or social worker. This should be routine. When we reject a 'disease model' of care and adopt a 'human-centred' model, the law relating to mental health could change significantly. There would be different criteria governing to whom the law applies, different ways of assuring that people are offered care that is (in the words of the current law) 'least restrictive', with a psychosocial focus, new roles for new professions, and a greater focus on social justice and judicial oversight.

## Article 6: mental health teams need to be radically different

Teams should be multidisciplinary, democratic and based on a psycho-social model. A psychosocial approach to service delivery would mean increased investment in the full range of professionals able to deliver these therapeutic services. Peer professionals, namely people with lived experience of mental health problems, will be particularly valuable, as will those skilled in practical issues such as finding employment or training. In the multidisciplinary teams delivering these services, psychiatric colleagues will remain valuable colleagues. An ideal model for interdisciplinary working would see leadership of such teams determined by the skills and personal qualities of the individual members of the team, rather than by their profession. It would not be assumed that medical colleagues should have 'clinical primacy' or unquestioned authority.

## Article 7: mental health services should be under local authority control

Mental health services should be based in local authorities, alongside other social, community-based, services. The thrust of the arguments in this book culminates in a simple message. The psychological, emotional and behavioural problems that are commonly referred to as mental health problems are fundamentally social and psychological issues. Psychologists, therapists and social workers must work closely alongside GPs, public health physicians, nurses and psychiatrists. But mental health and well-being is fundamentally a psychological and social phenomenon, with medical aspects. It is not, fundamentally, a medical phenomenon with additional psychological and social elements. It follows that the correct place for mental health care is within the social care system.

That doesn't mean that we should design medical teams for psychiatry, and manage them out of hospital-based, NHS-based Trusts but, instead, housed in a building away from the hospital site as a gesture to being 'community-based'. It means that we should locate the whole service in the community – put it entirely under local authority control. In the UK, we have the model of public health, recently transferred to local authority control, to build upon. Such services should be – and could then be – under democratic local governance.

## Article 8: we must establish the social prerequisites for genuine mental health and well-being

Our mental health and well-being are largely dependent on our social circumstances. To promote genuine mental health and well-being we need to protect and promote universal human rights, as enshrined in the United Nations' Universal Declaration of Human Rights. Because experiences of neglect, rejection and abuse are hugely important in the genesis of many problems, we need to redouble our efforts to protect children from emotional, physical or sexual abuse and neglect. Equally, we must protect both adults and children from bullying and discrimination: whether that is racism, homophobia, or discrimination based on sexuality, gender, disability or 'mental health' or any other characteristic. We can all do more to combat discrimination and promote a more tolerant and accepting society. More generally, if we are serious about preventing mental health problems from developing, and about promoting genuine psychological well-being, we must work collectively to create a more humane society: to reduce or eliminate poverty, especially childhood poverty, and to reduce financial and social inequality. We need to work harder to promote peace, social justice and equity, and ensure that citizens are properly fed, housed, and educated, and living in a sustainable natural ecosystem. We need to promote social mobility and social inclusion, encourage actions aimed at the common or collective good (for instance through practical support of local charitable activities), and reduce both corruption and materialistic greed. In a fair society, in a society that protects our mental health and well-being, we would ensure that everyone had a meaningful job or role in society and we would eliminate unhealthy organisational cultures at work.

Adopting this approach would result in a transfer of mental health services from the health to social services management (including a shift from hospital to residential care); a substantial reduction in the prescription of medication; a shift of medical responsibility from psychiatry to GPs with commensurate reduction in psychiatrist numbers; and the training or retraining of a large number of current workers in mental health care in a psychosocial approach.

This would require much greater emphasis on, training in, and staffing of, psychosocial approaches, and would represent a very major revolution in mental health services and in psychiatric practice. It would challenge the central tenets of at least some traditionalist, biological psychiatrists and the implications could be significant as their power and authority is challenged.

Nevertheless these proposals would be entirely affordable, and may even liberate resources for greater investment in mental health and well-being.

# Notes

## Introduction: The Disease Model of Mental Health: A System in Crisis

1. http://www.jacquidillon.org/biography/
2. D.E. Bloom, E.T. Cafiero, E. Jané-Llopis, S. Abrahams-Gessel, L.R. Bloom, S. Fathima, A.B. Feigl, T. Gaziano, M. Mowafi, A. Pandya, K. Prettner, L. Rosenberg, B. Seligman, A.Z. Stein and C. Weinstein (2011) *The Global Economic Burden of Noncommunicable Diseases*, Geneva: World Economic Forum.
3. Division of Clinical Psychology (2013) *Division of Clinical Psychology Position Statement on the Classification of Behaviour and Experience in Relation to Functional Psychiatric Diagnoses*, Leicester: British Psychological Society.
4. http://speakoutagainstpsychiatry.org/how-to-escape-from-a-psychiatric-hospital/
5. D.L. Rosenhan (1973) On Being Sane in Insane Places. *Science*, 179(4070): 250–8. PMID 4683124.
6. http://www.guardian.co.uk/news/datablog/2012/may/02/uk-healthcare-spending-gdp
7. http://www.schizophreniacommission.org.uk/the-report/
8. http://www.nice.org.uk/cg136
9. http://www.cqc.org.uk/public/reports-surveys-and-reviews/surveys/inpatient-survey-2013
10. http://www.guardian.co.uk/society/2006/oct/25/mentalhealth.socialcare
11. http://www.ohchr.org/Documents/HRBodies/HRCouncil/RegularSession/Session22/A.HRC.22.53_English.pdf
12. http://www.forbes.com/sites/emilywillingham/2013/03/08/autism-shock-therapy-is-torture-says-un-official/
13. Jablensky, N. Sartorius, G. Ernberg, M. Anker, A. Korten, J.E. Cooper, R. Day and A. Bertelsen (1992) *Schizophrenia: Manifestations, Incidence and Course in Different Cultures. A World Health Organization Ten-Country Study*. Psychological Medicine Monograph Supplement 20. Cambridge: Cambridge University Press. This paper and its implications are discussed in greater length in James Davies' excellent book detailed in Note 15.
14. http://www.guardian.co.uk/news/datablog/2012/may/02/uk-healthcare-spending-gdp
15. For an excellent description of this process in effect, see chapter 10 of J. Davies (2013) *Cracked: Why Psychiatry is Doing More Harm Than Good*, London: Icon Press. ISBN 9781848315563.
16. J. Joseph and C. Ratner (2013) 'The Fruitless Search For Genes In Psychiatry And Psychology: Time To Reexamine A Paradigm', in S. Krimsky, J. Gruber, R Hubbard, S. Newman, E.F. Keller (eds), *Genetic Explanations: Sense And Nonsense*, Massachusetts: Harvard University Press. ISBN 9780674064461.
17. J. Read, R. Fosse, A. Moskowitz and B. Perry (2014) The Traumagenic Neurodevelopmental Model of Psychosis Revisited. *Neuropsychiatry*, 4(1): 65–79. doi:10.2217/npy.13.89

18. D. Bhugra (1989) Attitudes Towards Mental Illness: A Review of the Literature. *Acta Psychiatrica Scandinavica*. 80(1): 1–12. DOI: 10.1111/j.1600–0447.1989. tb01293.x
19. J. Read, N. Haslam, L. Sayce and E. Davies (2006) Prejudice and Schizophrenia: A Review of the "Mental Illness is an Illness Like Any Other" Approach. *Acta Psychiatrica Scandinavica*, 114: 303–318. 10.1111/j.1600–0447.2006.00824.x
20. S. Mehta and A. Farina (1997) Is Being 'Sick' Really Better? The Effect of the Disease View of Mental Disorder on Stigma. *Journal of Social and Clinical Psychology*, 16: 405–419; and J. Read and N. Harré (2001) The Role of Biological and Genetic Causal Beliefs in the Stigmatisation of 'Mental Patients. *Journal of Mental Health*, 10(2): 223–235. doi:10.1080/09638230123129.
21. J. Read and R.P. Bentall (2012) Negative Childhood Experiences and Mental Health: Theoretical, Clinical and Primary Prevention Implications. *The British Journal of Psychiatry*, 200: 89–91; doi: 10.1192/bjp.bp.111.096727 and F. Varese, F. Smeets, M. Drukker, R. Lieverse, T. Lataster, W. Viechtbauer, J. Read, J. van Os and R.P. Bentall (2012) Childhood Adversities Increase the Risk of Psychosis: A Meta-analysis of Patient-Control, Prospective- and Cross-sectional Cohort Studies. *Schizophrenia Bulletin*, doi: 10.1093/schbul/sbs050
22. R. Wilkinson and K. Pickett (2009) *The Spirit Level: Why More Equal Societies Almost Always Do Better*, London: Allen Lane. ISBN 9780241954294. The associated website provides some useful information as well – www.equalitytrust.org.uk
23. L. Sideli, A. Mule, D. La Barbera and R.M. Murray (2012) Do Child Abuse and Maltreatment Increase Risk of Schizophrenia? *Psychiatry Investigation*, 9(2): 87–99.
24. N.M. Williams, I. Zaharieva, A. Martin, K. Langley, K. Mantripragada, R. Fossdal, H. Stefansson, K. Stefansson, P. Magnusson, O.O. Gudmundsson, O. Gustafsson, P. Holmans, M.J. Owen, M. O'Donovan and A. Thapar (2010) Rare Chromosomal Deletions and Duplications in Attention Deficit Hyperactivity Disorder: A Genome-wide Analysis. *Lancet*, 376(9750): 1401–1408.
25. http://www.badscience.net/2010/10/pride-and-prejudice/
26. www.nimh.nih.gov/about/director/2013/transforming-diagnosis.shtml
27. J. Moncrieff (2013) *The Bitterest Pills. The Troubling Story of Antipsychotic Drugs*, London: Palgrave Macmillan. ISBN 9781137277435.
28. For detailed discussion of all these issues, see R. Bentall (2009) *Doctoring the Mind: Why Psychiatric Treatments Fail*, London: Allen Lane. ISBN 9780141023694; and R. Whitaker (2010) *Anatomy of an Epidemic: Magic Bullets, Psychiatric Drugs, and the Astonishing Rise of Mental Illness in America*, New York: Crown (Random House). ISBN 9780307452412.
29. See Note 27 above, but also J. Moncrieff (2009) *The Myth of the Chemical Cure: A Critique of Psychiatric Drug Treatment*, London: Palgrave Macmillan. ISBN 9780230574328.
30. http://www.cqc.org.uk/sites/default/files/documents/cqc_mentalhealth_2012_13_07_update.pdf
31. For more information on the history of psychiatry, try reading: R. Porter (2002) *Madness: A Brief History*, Oxford: Oxford University Press. ISBN 0192802666; or E. Shorter (1997) *A History of Psychiatry: From the Era of the Asylum to the Age of Prozac*, New York: John Wiley & Sons, Inc. ISBN 9780471245315.

32. National Institute for Mental Health in England (2004) *Guidance on New Ways of Working for Psychiatrists in a Multidisciplinary and Multi-agency Context*, National Institute of Mental Health in England. London.
33. P. Bracken, P. Thomas, S. Timimi, E. Asen, G. Behr, C. Beuster, S. Bhunnoo, I. Browne, N. Chhina, D. Double, S. Downer, C. Evans, S. Fernando, M.R. Garland, W. Hopkins, R. Huws, B. Johnson, B. Martindale, H. Middleton, D. Moldavsky, J. Moncrieff, S. Mullins, J. Nelki, M. Pizzo, J. Rodger, M. Smyth, D. Summerfield, J. Wallace, D. Yeomans, D. (2012) Psychiatry beyond the Current Paradigm. *British Journal of Psychiatry*, 201(6): 430–434. doi: 10.1192/bjp.bp.112.109447
34. N. Craddock, D. Antebi, M.J. Attenburrow, A. Bailey, A. Carson, P. Cowen, B. Craddock, J. Eagles, K. Ebmeier, A. Farmer, S. Fazel, N. Ferrier, J. Geddes, G. Goodwin, P. Harrison, K. Hawton, S. Hunter, R. Jacoby, I. Jones, P. Keedwell, M. Kerr, P. Mackin, P. McGuffin, D.J. Macintyre, P. McConville, D. Mountain, M.C. O'Donovan, M.J. Owen, F. Oyebode, M. Phillips, J. Price, P. Shah, D.J. Smith, J. Walters, P. Woodruff, A. Young and S. Zammit (2008) Wake-up Call for British Psychiatry. *British Journal of Psychiatry*, 193(1): 6–9.
35. http://www.theguardian.com/society/2013/nov/27/dinesh-bhugra-psychiatry-mental-illness
36. See note 32 above.
37. P. Kinderman (2014) *New Laws of Psychology: Why Nature and Nurture Alone Cannot Explain Human Behaviour*, London: Constable and Robinson. ISBN 9781780336008.
38. http://www.soterianetwork.org.uk

# 1 Get the Message Right: A Psychosocial Model of Mental Health and Well-being

1. R.P. Bentall (2003) *Madness Explained: Psychosis and Human Nature*, London: Allen Lane. ISBN 9780140275407.
2. S.B. Guze (1989) Biological Psychiatry: Is there Any Other Kind? *Psychological Medicine*, 19: 315–323.
3. E.R. Kandel (1998) A New Intellectual Framework for Psychiatry. *American Journal of Psychiatry*, 155: 457–468.
4. See footnote 27 in earlier chapter – N. Craddock, D. Antebi, M.J. Attenburrow, A. Bailey, A. Carson, P. Cowen, B. Craddock, J. Eagles, K. Ebmeier, A. Farmer, S. Fazel, N. Ferrier, J. Geddes, G. Goodwin, P. Harrison, K. Hawton, S. Hunter, R. Jacoby, I. Jones, P. Keedwell, M. Kerr, P. Mackin, P. McGuffin, D.J. Macintyre, P. McConville, D. Mountain, M.C. O'Donovan, M.J. Owen, F. Oyebode, M. Phillips, J. Price, P. Shah, D.J. Smith, J. Walters, P. Woodruff, A. Young, and S. Zammit (2008) Wake-up Call for British Psychiatry. *British Journal of Psychiatry*, 193(1): 6–9.
5. See footnote 26 in earlier chapter – P. Bracken, P. Thomas, S. Timimi, E. Asen, G. Behr, C. Beuster, S. Bhunnoo, I. Browne, N. Chhina, D. Double, S. Downer, C. Evans, S. Fernando, M.R. Garland, W. Hopkins, R. Huws, B. Johnson, B. Martindale, H. Middleton, D. Moldavsky, J. Moncrieff, S. Mullins, J. Nelki, M. Pizzo, J. Rodger, M. Smyth, D. Summerfield, J. Wallace, and D. Yeomans (2012) Psychiatry Beyond the Current Paradigm. *British Journal of Psychiatry*, 201(6): 430–434. doi: 10.1192/bjp.bp.112.109447

6. See footnote 25 in earlier chapter – National Institute for Mental Health in England (2004) Guidance on New Ways of Working for Psychiatrists in a Multi-disciplinary and Multi-agency Context. *National Institute for Mental Health in England*. London.
7. http://www.iapt.nhs.uk/silo/files/iapt-3-year-report.pdf (see page 18)
8. R. Wilkinson, and K. Pickett (2009) The Spirit Level: Why More Equal Societies Almost Always Do Better, London: Allen Lane. ISBN 9780241954294. See also www.equalitytrust.org.uk.
9. B. Barr, D. Taylor-Robinson, A. Scott-Samuel, M. McKee, and D. Stuckler (2012) Suicides Associated with the 2008–2010 Economic Recession in England: Time Trend Analysis, *British Medical Journal*, 345: e5142. See also http://www.bmj.com/content/345/bmj.e5142.
10. See footnote 20 in earlier chapter: L. Sideli, A. Mule, D. La Barbera, and R.M. Murray (2012) Do Child Abuse and Maltreatment Increase Risk of Schizophrenia? *Psychiatry Investigation*, 9(2): 87–99.
11. P. Kinderman (2005) A Psychological Model of Mental Disorder, *Harvard Review of Psychiatry*, 13: 206–217.

# 2   Understand, Don't Diagnose

1. P. Kinderman, E. Setzu, F. Lobban and P. Salmon (2006) Illness Beliefs in Schizophrenia. *Social Science and Medicine*, 63: 1900–1911. doi: 10.1016/j.socscimed.2006.04.022.
2. Richard Bentall discusses the historical background to psychiatric diagnosis in his book 'Madness Explained', which I cited in Chapter 1, Note 1; R.P. Bentall (2003) *Madness Explained: Psychosis and Human Nature*, London: Allen Lane. ISBN 9780140275407.
3. http://www.mind.org.uk/information-support/types-of-mental-health-problems/statistics-and-facts-about-mental-health/how-common-are-mental-health-problems/
4. ICD-10 is described well on the WHO website: www.who.int/classifications/icd/en/ The full reference is: World Health Organization (1992) *International Statistical Classification of Diseases and Related Health Problems*, Geneva: World Health Organization.
5. American Psychiatric Association (2013) *Diagnostic and Statistical Manual of Mental Disorders*, 5th edn, Washington, DC: American Psychiatric Association.
6. Living with Grief. *The Lancet* (Editorial), 2012: 379.
7. World Health Organization, (1973) *The International Pilot Study of Schizophrenia*, Geneva: World Health Organization; and World Health Organization, (1979) *Schizophrenia: An International Follow-up Study*, New York: Wiley.
8. There is an excellent on-line article by Jack Carney on the declining reliability statistics for the DSM franchise: http://www.madinamerica.com/2013/03/the-dsm-5-field-trials-inter-rater-reliability-ratings-take-a-nose-dive/
9. Any such laboratory tests might well be largely meaningless even if they existed, because depression and other mental health issues are essentially problems of experience, not biology. If you were to be experiencing major problems, a negative test result would still leave you with problems, and

they'd need to be addressed. A positive test would tell you nothing more than you already knew, although it might offer spurious scientific confirmation. If you had no significant problems but 'tested positive', I doubt that you would accept a prescription for antidepressants (or therapy)...at least until you started experiencing difficulties, when my first point would apply. There's an interesting, if slightly densely written, historical account of these issues in this paper: R. Noll, (2006) The Blood of the Insane. *History of Psychiatry*, 17(4): 395–418 DOI: 10.1177/0957154X06059440 or http://peer. ccsd.cnrs.fr/docs/00/57/08/43/PDF/PEER_stage2_10.1177%252F0957154X0 6059440.pdf

10. Cartwright set out his ideas in a journal article: Report on the Diseases and Physical Peculiarities of the Negro Race. *The New Orleans Medical and Surgical Journal*, 1851: 691–715. A modern discussion of this idea can be found in: A.L. Caplan, J.J. McCartney and D.A. Sisti (eds) (2004) *Health, Disease, and Illness: Concepts in Medicine*, Washington: Georgetown University Press.

11. P. Kinderman, J. Read, J. Moncrieff and R.P. Bentall (2013) Drop the Language of Disorder. *Evidence Based Mental Health*, 16: 2–3. doi:10.1136/eb-2012–100987

12. D.L. Rosenhan (1973) On Being Sane in Insane Places. *Science*, 179(4070): 250–258. PMID 4683124.

13. Cross-Disorder Group of the Psychiatric Genomics Consortium (2013) Identification of Risk Loci with Shared Effects on Five Major Psychiatric Disorders: A Genome-wide Analysis. *The Lancet*, 381(9875): 1371–1379. doi:10.1016/S0140–6736(12)62129–1

14. Billy Budd is now out of copyright and freely available on the internet, for instance at: http://www2.hn.psu.edu/faculty/jmanis/melville/billy-budd.pdf

15. The *Times* is, remarkably, searchable online from as early as 1785. The Editorial quoted is for Saturday, 22 July 1854, p. 8.

16. S. Timimi (2005) *Naughty Boys: Anti-social Behaviour, ADHD and the Role of Culture*, London: Palgrave Macmillan. ISBN 9781403945112; S. Timimi, N. Gardner and B. McCabe (2010) *The Myth of Autism: Medicalising Men's and Boys' Social and Emotional Competence*, London: Palgrave Macmillan. ISBN 9780230545267.

17. See Notes 5 and 10 above as well as the 'Mad in America' website: http://www.madinamerica.com/

18. This is from 'Discursive of Tunbridge Wells', an excellent blog site addressing some of the same issues I discuss in this book. http://discursiveoftun-bridgewells.blogspot.co.uk/2014/01/flo-bellamy-does-diagnosis-simply.html

19. Gemma's thesis is available for public access but, unfortunately, only from the University of Liverpool Library, where it is lodged with the accession number: lvp.b2182260. I hope Gemma will publish her research in a journal article very soon.

20. J. Read and R.P. Bentall (2012) Negative Childhood Experiences and Mental Health: Theoretical, Clinical and Primary Prevention Implications. *British Journal of Psychiatry*, 200: 89–91.

21. As mentioned in Note 18, Fay writes for Discursive of Tunbridge Wells: http://discursiveoftunbridgewells.blogspot.co.uk/2013/09/the-lament-of-black-swan-i-dont-need-my.html

## 3   The Drugs Don't Work ... So Offer Real Solutions

1. Previously cited as Note 2 in the introductory chapter: D.E. Bloom, E.T. Cafiero, E. Jané-Llopis S. Abrahams-Gessel, L.R. Bloom, S. Fathima, A.B. Feigl, T. Gaziano, M. Mowafi, A. Pandya, K. Prettner, L. Rosenberg, B. Seligman, A.Z. Stein and C. Weinstein (2011) *The Global Economic Burden of Noncommunicable Diseases*, Geneva: World Economic Forum.
2. Department of Health (2011) *No Health Without Mental Health: A Cross-government Mental Health Outcomes Strategy for People of all Ages*, London: Department of Health. http://www.dh.gov.uk/en/Publicationsandstatistics/Publications/PublicationsPolicyAndGuidance/DH_123766
3. Hansard, the record of the UK Parliament, is available online. This particular debate is at: http://www.publications.parliament.uk/pa/cm201213/cmhansrd/cm120614/debtext/120614–0003.htm
4. http://bjp.rcpsych.org/content/200/5/393.long
5. J. Moncrieff (2013) *The Bitterest Pills. The Troubling Story of Antipsychotic Drugs*, London: Palgrave Macmillan.
6. http://joannamoncrieff.com
7. http://joannamoncrieff.com/2013/11/27/why-theres-no-such-thing-as-an-antidepressant/
8. J. Moncrieff and I. Kirsch (2005) Efficacy of Antidepressants in Adults. *British Medical Journal*, 331: 155–157. doi:10.1136/bmj.331.7509.155.
9. http://www.badscience.net
10. W. Moody, P. Kinderman and P. Sinha (2010) An Exploratory Study: Relationships between Trying on Clothing, Mood, Emotion, Personality and Clothing Preference. *Journal of Fashion Marketing and Management*, 14(1): 161–179. http://www.emeraldinsight.com/journals.htm?articleid=1840473
11. J. Moncrieff (2009) *The Myth of the Chemical Cure: A Critique of Psychiatric Drug Treatment*, London: Palgrave Macmillan. ISBN 9780230574328.
12. http://joannamoncrieff.com/2013/12/09/long-term-antipsychotics-making-sense-of-the-evidence/
13. P. Deniker (1960) Experimental Neurological Syndromes and the New Drug Therapies in Psychiatry. *Comprehensive Psychiatry*, 1: 92–102.
14. National Clinical Guideline Number 178. Psychosis and Schizophrenia in Adults: Treatment and Management. issued: February 2014, last modified: March 2014. London: National Institute for Health & Care Excellence. http://www.nice.org.uk/nicemedia/live/14382/66534/66534.pdf
15. See R. Bentall (2009) *Doctoring the Mind: Why Psychiatric Treatments Fail*, London: Allen Lane. ISBN 9780141023694; R. Whitaker (2010) *Anatomy of an Epidemic: Magic Bullets, Psychiatric Drugs, and the Astonishing Rise of Mental Illness in America*, New York: Crown (Random House) ISBN 978-0-307-45241-2; and J. Moncrieff (2013) *The Bitterest Pills. The Troubling Story of Antipsychotic Drugs*, London: Palgrave Macmillan. ISBN 9781137277435.
16. S.H. Jones, F. Lobban, A. Cooke, et al. (2010) *Understanding Bipolar Disorder: Why Some People Experience Extreme Mood States and What Can Help*, Leicester: British Psychological Society. http://www.psychminded.co.uk/news/news2010/October10/Understanding-bipolar-disorder.pdf
17. See Note 11.

18. Don't Keep Taking the Tablets. *British Medical Journal*, 2013; 347 doi: http://dx.doi.org/10.1136/bmj.f7438
19. M. McCarthy (2013) Antidepressant Use Has Doubled in Rich Nations in Past 10 Years. *British Medical Journal*, 347: f7261. doi:10.1136/bmj.f7261
20. C. Dowrick and A. Frances (2013) Medicalising Unhappiness: New Classification of Depression Risks More Patients Being Put on Drug Treatment From Which They Will Not Benefit. *British Medical Journal*, 347: f7140. doi:10.1136/bmj.f7140
21. See also Note 14 of Chapter 3: J. Davies (2013) *Cracked: Why Psychiatry is Doing More Harm Than Good*, London: Icon Press. ISBN 9781848315563.
22. S. Zisook, S.R. Shuchter, P. Pedrelli, J. Sable and S.C. Deaciuc (2001) Bupropion Sustained Release for Bereavement: Results of an Open Trial. *Journal of Clinical Psychiatry*, 62(4): 227–230. http://www.ncbi.nlm.nih.gov/pubmed/11379835
23. See Note 12
24. See, for instance M.M. Linehan (1995) Combining Pharmacotherapy with Psychotherapy for Substance Abusers with Borderline Personality Disorder: Strategies for Enhancing Compliance. NIDA Research Monograph Series: Integrating Behavioral Therapies with Medications in the Treatment of Drug Dependence, pp. 129–142, Rockville, MD: National Institute of Health.
25. http://www.candi.nhs.uk/services/services/drayton-park-womens-crisis-service/
26. A. Morrison, D. Turkington, M. Pyle, H. Spencer, A. Brabban, G. Dunn, T. Christodoulides, R. Dudley, N. Chapman, P. Callcott, T. Grace, V. Lumley, L. Drage, S. Tully, K. Irving, A. Cummings, R. Byrne, L.M. Davies and P. Hutton (2014) Cognitive Therapy for People with Schizophrenia Spectrum Disorders Not Taking Antipsychotic Drugs: A Single–Blind Randomised Controlled Trial. *The Lancet*. doi:10.1016/S0140–6736(13)62246–1
27. See also Note 30 in the introductory chapter; http://www.soterianetwork.org.uk
28. See, for example, the work at the Spectrum Centre at the University of Lancaster in the UK: www.lancaster.ac.uk/shm/research/spectrum/

# 4   Promote Health and Well-being

1. See: http://en.wikipedia.org/wiki/Social_pedagogy
2. World Health Organization (1948) Constitution of the World Health Organization, Geneva: World Health Organization. www.who.int/governance/eb/who_constitution_en.pdf
3. European Commission (2005) *Promoting the Mental Health of the Population. Towards a Strategy on Mental Health for the European Union*, Brussels: European Commission.
4. See earlier notes and Department of Health (2011) *No Health Without Mental Health: A Cross-Government Mental Health Outcomes Strategy for People of All Ages*, London: Department of Health. http://www.dh.gov.uk/en/Publicationsandstatistics/Publications/PublicationsPolicyAndGuidance/DH_123766
5. See also Note 7 in Chapter 1; B. Barr, D. Taylor-Robinson, A. Scott-Samuel, M. McKee and D. Stuckler (2012) Suicides Associated with the 2008–2010

Economic Recession in England: Time Trend Analysis. *British Medical Journal*, 345: e5142. http://www.bmj.com/content/345/bmj.e5142

6. A key report from the new economics foundation – www.nationalaccountsofwellbeing.org/ – describes these issues well: J. Michaelson, S. Abdallah, N. Steuer, S. Thompson and N. Marks, with J. Aked, C. Cordon and R. Potts (2009) *National Accounts of Well-being: Bringing Real Wealth Onto the Balance Sheet*, London: New Economics Foundation.

7. R. Wilkinson and K. Pickett (2009) *The Spirit Level: Why More Equal Societies Almost Always Do Better*, London: Allen Lane. ISBN 9780241954294. See also www.equalitytrust.org.uk

8. World Health Organization (2003) *Social Determinants of Health: The Solid Facts*. 2nd edn (eds R. Wilkinson and M. Marmot), Geneva: World Health Organization. ISBN 9289013710.

9. P. Kinderman, M. Schwannauer, E. Pontin and S. Tai (2013) Psychological Processes Mediate the Impact of Familial Risk, Social Circumstances and Life Events on Mental Health. *PLoS ONE*, 8(10): e76564. http://dx.plos.org/10.1371/journal.pone.0076564.

10. http://www.bbc.co.uk/news/magazine-24444431

11. For personal advice, see: http://www.nhs.uk/livewell/Pages/Livewellhub.aspx

12. The Five Ways to Wellbeing is a set of evidence-based public mental health messages developed by the new economics foundation as part of the Foresight Project on Mental Capital and Wellbeing: http://www.neweconomics.org/publications/entry/five-ways-to-well-being-the-evidence. Many NHS Trusts and local authorities, including the City of Liverpool, have adopted the Five Ways message: www.2010healthandwellbeing.org.uk/. The full academic reference to the Five Ways to Wellbeing is: J. Aked and S. Thompson (2011) *Five Ways to Wellbeing: New Applications, New Ways of Thinking*. London: New Economic Foundation.

13. The Reader Organisation – www.thereader.org.uk

14. J. Kabat-Zinn (1994) *Wherever You Go, There You Are: Mindfulness Meditation for Everyday Life*, London: Piatkus. ISBN 9780749925482.

15. P. Kinderman (1994) Cognitive Behaviour Therapy for Depression in the Year 1411. *Clinical Psychology & Psychotherapy*, 1: 116–119.

16. www.nice.org.uk/

17. This press release is surprisingly difficult to find online. The original release had the URL of http://www.dh.gov.uk/en/Publicationsandstatistics/pressreleases/DH_4134785 but this has been taken off the Department of Health's website. The release can be found at: http://webarchive.nationalarchives.gov.uk/20060522092154/http://www.dh.gov.uk/PublicationsAndStatistics/PressReleases/PressReleasesNotices/fs/en?CONTENT_ID=4134785&chk=HKLLdo

18. http://www.theguardian.com/society/2005/oct/11/mentalhealth.socialcare

19. P. Kinderman (2014) *New Laws of Psychology: Why Nature and Nurture Alone Cannot Explain Human Behaviour*, Constable and Robinson, London. ISBN 9781780336008.

20. The ICS or interacting cognitive subsystems model is a very technical, frankly complicated, psychological theory of how our thoughts work. But although it's complicated, it's also brilliant. Probably the easiest to

read paper is: P.J. Barnard and J.D. Teasdale (1991) Interacting Cognitive Subsystems: A Systemic Approach to Cognitive–Affective Interaction and Change. *Cognition and Emotion*, 5: 1–39. http://www.tandfonline.com/doi/abs/10.1080/02699939108411021

21. Many psychologists have studied change blindness. Christopher Chabris and Daniel Simons are responsible for the 'invisible gorilla' effect, and have used this engaging approach to good effect on their website www.theinvisible-gorilla.com/videos.html and in print: C. Chabris and D. Simons (2011) *The Invisible Gorilla: How Our Intuitions Deceive Us*, New York: Broadway.

22. D. Kahneman, P. Slovic and A. Tversky (1982) *Judgment Under Uncertainty: Heuristics and Biases*, New York: Cambridge University Press. ISBN: 0521284147

23. http://www.iapt.nhs.uk/silo/files/talking-therapies-a-four-year-plan-of-action.pdf

# 5 Residential Care ... Not Medical Coercion

1. The Act can be read here: http://www.legislation.gov.uk/ukpga/2007/12/contents but it is quite complex and legalistic. The Wikipedia page is, therefore, helpful: http://en.wikipedia.org/wiki/Mental_Health_Act_2007

2. http://www.rcpsych.ac.uk/pdf/NAS%20National%20report%20FINAL.pdf

3. http://www.rcpsych.ac.uk/files/pdfversion/op67.pdf

4. See earlier footnotes and Department of Health (2011) *No Health Without Mental Health: A Cross-government Mental Health Outcomes Strategy for People of all Ages*, London: Department of Health. http://www.dh.gov.uk/en/Publicationsandstatistics/Publications/PublicationsPolicyAndGuidance/DH_123766sd

5. I.M. Hunt, K. Windfuhr, J. Shaw, L. Appleby and N. Kapur (2012) Ligature Points and Ligature Types Used by Psychiatric In-patients Who Die by Hanging: A National Study. *Crisis: The Journal of Crisis Intervention and Suicide Prevention*, 33: 87–94. http://www.ncbi.nlm.nih.gov/pubmed/22343063

6. http://www.guardian.co.uk/commentisfree/2013/feb/01/mental-health-services-coercion

7. http://www.asylumonline.net/too-much-coercion-in-mental-health-services-by-richard-bentall/

8. Intelligent reviews of mental health legislation can be found in: J. Bindman, S. Maingay and G. Szmukler (2003) The Human Rights Act and Mental Health Legislation. *British Journal of Psychiatry*, 182: 91–94; and G. Szmukler and F. Holloway (2000) Reform of the Mental Health Act. Health or Safety? *British Journal of Psychiatry*, 177: 196–200.

9. http://www.communitycare.co.uk/2008/11/11/mental-health-acts-1983-and-2007/#.UsQ-Gf0SjwI

10. The specific case involved (Winterwerp v. The Netherlands (Article 50) – 6301/73 [1981] ECHR 7 (27 November 1981)) is discussed in: M.L. Perlin, K. Gledhill, M.P. Treuthart, E. Szeli and A. Kanter (2006) *International Human Rights and Comparative Mental Disability Law: Cases and Materials*, Durham, NC: Carolina Academic Press.

11. http://www.legislation.gov.uk/asp/2003/13/contents

12. D. Smail (1993) Putting Our Mouths Where Our Money Is. *Clinical Psychology Forum*, 61: 11–14.

# 6  Teamworking

1. P. Kinderman, W. Sellwood and S. Tai (2007) Policy Implications of a Psychological Model of Mental Disorder', *Journal of Mental Health*. 17(1): 93–103. DOI: 10.1080/09638230701530226
2. J. Van Os, C.M. Gilvarry, R. Bale, E. Van Horn and T. Tattan (1998) Assessment of Psychopathological Dimensions Improves Clinical Reasoning. *Schizophrenia Research*, 29(1–2): 40.
3. A. Cooke, (ed.) (2014) 'Understanding 'Psychosis' and 'Schizophrenia': Why people sometimes hear voices, believe things that others find strange, or appear out of touch with reality, and what can help'. A report by the British Psychological Society Division of Clinical Psychology. Leicester: British Psychological. Available from www.understandingpsychosis.net
4. P. Kinderman (2002) The Future of Clinical Psychology Training. *Clinical Psychology*, 8: 6–10.
5. R. Warner (1994) *Recovery from Schizophrenia: Psychiatry and Political Economy* (2nd edn). Routledge: New York.
6. Care Services Improvement Partnership & National Institute for Mental Health in England (2006) *The Social Work Contribution to Mental Health Services – The Future Direction*. London: Care Services Improvement Partnership & National Institute for Mental Health in England.
7. See http://www.rywu.org.uk/wp-content/uploads/2010/05/Social-Pedagogy-Report.pdf as well as J. Kornbeck (2002) Reflections on the Exportability of Social Pedagogy and its Possible Limits. *Social Work in Europe*, 9(2): 37–49; and S. Asquith, C. Clark and L. Waterhouse (2005) *The Scottish Review of the Future of Social Work* http://www.scotland.gov.uk/Resource/Doc/47121/0020821.pdf
8. Department of Health (2006) *From Values to Action: The Chief Nursing Officer's Review of Mental Health Nursing*, London: Department of Health.
9. S. Lancashire, G. Haddock, N. Tarrier, I. Baguley, A.C. Butterworth and C. Brooker (1997) Effects of Training in Psychosocial Interventions for Community Psychiatric Nurses in England. *Psychiatric Services*, 48(1): 39–41.
10. J. Boardman, B. Grove, R. Perkins and G. Shepherd (2003) Work and Employment for People with Psychiatric Disabilities. *British Journal of Psychiatry*, 182: 467–468.
11. P. Huxley and G. Thornicroft (2003) Social Inclusion, Social Quality and Mental Illness. *British Journal of Psychiatry*, 182: 289–290; Office of the Deputy Prime Minister (2004) *Mental Health and Social Exclusion: Social Exclusion Unit Report*, London: Office of the Deputy Prime Minister.
12. National Institute for Mental Health in England (2004) *Guidance on New Ways of Working for Psychiatrists in a Multi-disciplinary and Multi-agency Context*, London: National Institute of Mental Health in England.
13. A. Haunstein Swan (2005) Lessons I learned in War Zones. *Clinical Psychology*, 46: 6–9.

# 7  Social and Community Services in Local Authority Management

1. P. Bracken, P. Thomas, S. Timimi, E. Asen, G. Behr, C. Beuster, S. Bhunnoo, I. Browne, N. Chhina, D. Double, S. Downer, C. Evans, S. Fernando, M.R.

Garland, W. Hopkins, R. Huws, B. Johnson, B. Martindale, H. Middleton, D. Moldavsky, J. Moncrieff, S. Mullins, J. Nelki, M. Pizzo, J. Rodger, M. Smyth, D. Summerfield, J. Wallace and D. Yeomans (2012) Psychiatry Beyond the Current Paradigm. *British Journal of Psychiatry*, 201(6): 430–434. doi: 10.1192/bjp.bp.112.109447
2. http://www.legislation.gov.uk/ukpga/2012/7/contents/enacted    and    read about the controversies here: http://en.wikipedia.org/wiki/Health_and_Social_Care_Act_2012
3. http://www.bbc.co.uk/news/business-25240202

# 8  Can We Afford It?

1. As I mentioned in the previous chapter, Note 3, it seems to be a matter of pride to some in government that the UK is planning to return to a level of under-funding for public services not seen since 1948; http://www.bbc.co.uk/news/business-25240202
2. http://www.nhsconfed.org/priorities/political-engagement/Pages/NHS-statistics.aspx
3. http://eprints.lse.ac.uk/42050/1/How_the_NHS_measures_up_to_other_health_systems_(LSERO).pdf
4. http://webarchive.nationalarchives.gov.uk/20101111021302/http://www.nmhdu.org.uk/silo/files/nmhdu-factfile-3.pdf
5. see  https://www.gov.uk/government/publications/public-health-transitional-support-funds    and    https://www.gov.uk/government/uploads/system/uploads/attachment_data/file/212971/Transitional-Support-letter-LACE1.pdf
6. R. Layard (2005) Mental Health: Britain's Biggest Social Problem. Cabinet Office briefing paper. available at http://eprints.lse.ac.uk/47428/
7. Department of Health (2006) From Values to Action: The Chief Nursing Officer's Review of Mental Health Nursing. London: Department of Health, http://webarchive.nationalarchives.gov.uk/20060829080949/http://dh.gov.uk/prod_consum_dh/idcplg?IdcService=GET_FILE&dID=4368&Rendition=Web
8. All my figures date from 2010, represent 'full-time equivalents' and are available at: http://data.gov.uk/dataset/nhs-staff-2000–2010-non-medical
9. https://hee.nhs.uk/work-programmes/resources/
10. http://www.nhscareers.nhs.uk/working-in-the-nhs/pay-and-benefits/agenda-for-change-pay-rates/
11. http://www.bmj.com/content/344/bmj.e4250
12. http://www.nao.org.uk/wp-content/uploads/2006/05/05061041.pdf
13. www.bma.org.uk/press_centre/pressgps.jsp
14. www.rcpsych.ac.uk/pdf/2009%20Census.pdf
15. See previous Note; www.rcpsych.ac.uk/pdf/2009%20Census.pdf

# Index

Printed and bound by CPI Group (UK) Ltd, Croydon, CR0 4YY